ROUTLEDGE LIBRARY EDITIONS: HEALTH, DISEASE & SOCIETY

Volume 20

CHOLERA 1832

CHOLERA 1832

The Social Response to an Epidemic

R. J. MORRIS

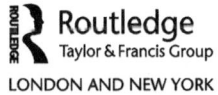

LONDON AND NEW YORK

First published in 1976 by Croom Helm Ltd.

This edition first published in 2022
by Routledge
4 Park Square, Milton Park, Abingdon, Oxon OX14 4RN

and by Routledge
605 Third Avenue, New York, NY 10158

Routledge is an imprint of the Taylor & Francis Group, an informa business

© 1976 R. J. Morris

All rights reserved. No part of this book may be reprinted or reproduced or utilised in any form or by any electronic, mechanical, or other means, now known or hereafter invented, including photocopying and recording, or in any information storage or retrieval system, without permission in writing from the publishers.

Trademark notice: Product or corporate names may be trademarks or registered trademarks, and are used only for identification and explanation without intent to infringe.

British Library Cataloguing in Publication Data
A catalogue record for this book is available from the British Library

ISBN: 978-0-367-52469-2 (Set)
ISBN: 978-1-032-24419-8 (Volume 20) (hbk)
ISBN: 978-1-032-24420-4 (Volume 20) (pbk)
ISBN: 978-1-003-27850-4 (Volume 20) (ebk)

DOI: 10.4324/9781003278504

Publisher's Note
The publisher has gone to great lengths to ensure the quality of this reprint but points out that some imperfections in the original copies may be apparent.

Disclaimer
The publisher has made every effort to trace copyright holders and would welcome correspondence from those they have been unable to trace.

CHOLERA 1832

The Social Response to An Epidemic

R. J. MORRIS

CROOM HELM LONDON

© 1976 by R. J. Morris

Croom Helm Ltd
2-10 St John's Road, London SW11

ISBN 0-85664-377-7

Printed and bound in Great Britain
by Redwood Burn Ltd, Trowbridge and Esher

CONTENTS

Acknowledgements		9
1	Prologue	11
2	Approach	21
3	Sunderland	39
4	Containment Fails	59
5	Victims	79
6	Class, Power and Cholera	95
7	Religion and Morals	129
8	Medicine and Science	159
9	Epilogue	197
10	Reflections	213
Select Bibliography		217
Index		222

TABLES

1	Cholera Deaths in Britain, 1831-1866	13
2	Crude Death Rate in England and Wales, 1846-56 and 1865-67	13
3	Month by Month Progress of Cholera, 1831-1832	75
4	Burial Rates in Glasgow and Edinburgh, 1827-1837	82
5	Impact of Cholera on the Population of Glasgow, 1832: Age Structure	83
6	The First 64 Cases in Sunderland	88
7	Newburn: Those who Died between 2 January and 4 February 1832	89
8	Manchester: The First 200 Cases	89
9	Oxford: 174 Cases	90
10	Cholera and Occupational Status 1831-1832	91
11	Cholera and Status in Sunderland and Manchester 1832	92
12	Tabular View, showing Connection between the Subjects of Attacks to Cholera	188
13	Cholera Deaths and Water Supplies in London	209

MAPS

1. Bengal to Sunderland, 1826-1831
2. England and Wales, 1831-1832
3. North-East England, Winter 1831-1832
4. Scotland 1831-1832
5. London 1832-1866

FIGURES

1. Age-specific Burial Rates and Age Structure of Glasgow, 1830-1831
2. Religion, Cholera and Social Status

ABBREVIATIONS

E.M.S.J.   *Edinburgh Medical and Surgical Journal*
C.O.   *Christian Observer*
W.M.M.   *Wesleyan Methodist Magazine*
P.P. (H. of C.) *British Parliamentary Papers,* House of Commons series
P.R.O.   Public Record Office, London

ACKNOWLEDGEMENTS

I first learnt of cholera in one of those stories my grandmother used to tell. Apparently a long-dead ancestor of mine had walked from central Wales to Liverpool during the epidemic of 1832. She had a spare pair of boots around her neck and did not trust the authorities to take proper care of another relative who was a cholera victim in the city. This study began as part of a larger examination of the middle class in nineteenth-century Leeds. The cholera of 1832 was an incident in the history of public health and class relationships in Leeds which seemed to require explanation in terms of the religious and scientific understanding of the people involved as well as those economic, political and class relationships which are the traditional concern of social historians. This led to an enquiry into the sociology of nineteenth-century scientific thought, religion and administration which went far beyond Leeds and its middle class.

I have received help and advice from many people during the course of researching and writing. Mr J.H. Collinson, the Leeds City Archivist, and Mrs G.C.F. Forster, the Honorary Librarian of the Thoresby Society, helped me in the early days. My work in Oxford was assisted by the staff of the Bodleian Library and the Secretary of the Radcliffe Infirmary, Oxford to whom I am grateful for giving me permission to see papers in his care. The staff of the National Library of Scotland cheerfully produced mountains of periodicals and pamphlets for me. My thanks to them for making Scotland such an enjoyable place to work in. The lines from 'The Dry Salvages' are reprinted by permission of Faber and Faber Ltd. from *The Four Quartets* by T.S. Eliot. Ailsa Maxwell, Hilary Turner, Michael Cullen, Roger Davidson, Derek Fraser, Sheridan Gilley, Michael Rose and Patrick Scott have all helped with sources or guided me through unfamiliar areas of historical literature. Betty Ewins did some preliminary research in the Public Record Office and thus helped make my trips to London much more productive. At various stages in research and writing I exchanged ideas with Alan MacLaren, Margaret Pelling and Mick Durey, three other scholards who have concerned themselves with nineteenth-century cholera. A discussion with Father Noel O'Donoghue of New College in Edinburgh greatly assisted my understanding of the attitudes of the Catholic parish priest, though I am not sure how far he would agree with the conclusions I came to in the book. Professor M.W. Flinn, Dr N.T. Phillipson and Professor T.C. Smout all read an earlier version of the manuscript and made many helpful comments. Dr A.G. Leitch of the Medical School in Edinburgh delivered a medical opinion on the 'body'. Professor John Harrison and Stephen Yeo gave valuable editorial help. My thanks to Fiona Douglas who with the assistance of Mrs Scott and Mrs Hunter, bore the brunt of the typing with so much enthusiasm. My greatest debt is to Barbara Morris, wife and cartographer, who drew the maps and provided large supplies of patience and encouragement to ease the path of research and writing. Even she could not curb those errors which may remain to my credit.

R.J. Morris
Edinburgh
February 1976

1 PROLOGUE

William Sproat, a keelman, of Sunderland, County Durham, began his short but disastrous contribution to British medical history on Sunday, 23 October 1831. On the Saturday, thinking he was recovering from a bad bout of summer diarrhoea, he had a mutton chop for dinner (much against his doctor's advice), and walked from his house near the Long Bank in Sunderland to his keel on the river. On his return, 'He became very ill, had a severe shivering fit and giddiness, cramps of the stomach, and violent vomiting and purging.' When Mr Holmes, his surgeon, was called on Sunday morning he found him:

> Evidently sinking; pulse almost imperceptible, and extremities cold, skin dry, eyes sunk, lips blue, features shrunk, he spoke in whispers, violent vomiting and purging, cramps of the calves and legs, and complete prostration of strength.

By mid-afternoon Sproat had been visited by two other doctors; Dr Clanny, one of the leaders of the local medical profession, and J.B. Kell, surgeon to the reserve units of the 82nd Regiment then stationed in Sunderland barracks. Kell was of little account in terms of local or professional status but he had seen and treated Asiatic cholera whilst stationed in Mauritius. He examined Sproat, confirmed that this was a case of Asiatic cholera, and Clanny agreed with his verdict. Holmes continued to visit Sproat regularly, but could do little more than attempt to restore his shattered circulation with a little brandy and hot bricks applied to the feet, and try to settle his stomach and pain with opium and calomel. On Wednesday, Holmes found his patient worse, 'Pulse scarcely beating under the fingers, countenance quite shrunken, lips dark blue. . .at twelve o'clock at noon he died.'

William Sproat was the first confirmed case of Asiatic cholera in the British Isles. It was certain that others had died in Sunderland during the late summer of 1831. But Kell and Clanny only gained hearsay knowledge of such cases, sometimes months afterwards. The doctors who saw them could not recognise the disease, and those who suspected something was wrong were reluctant to admit that cholera had arrived in Sunderland. Within a few days of Sproat's death, his son was dead and his grand-daughter was slowly recovering from the fever which followed in patients fortunate enough to survive the initial attack.[1]

These histories of collapse, pain and death were to be repeated many times throughout Britain over the next eighteen months. Britain was seriously affected by four of the pandemics of cholera which have spread from Bengal since the early nineteenth century; namely in 1831-2, in 1848-9, in 1853-4 and in 1866. After that cholera made no more than a few incursions in port and coastal areas. Figures of varying quality are available for each epidemic (Table 1). The Registrar-General's figures (England and Wales, 1848-9, 1853-4 and 1866, and Scotland 1866) are comparable and as accurate as possible; a few cases missed because doctors failed to recognise the disease, and other cases of English cholera included in the total. The other figures are all likely to be underestimated, especially in 1831-2, when failure to recognise the disease was a more serious problem and many places were reluctant to admit the presence of the disease for fear of disrupting trade or deterring visitors. Several places, like Yarmouth and Salisbury, failed to make any return at all. Only a small portion of these omissions was compensated for by doctors who attributed deaths from other bowel disorders to the Asiatic totals. These tables show deaths only. Recording of cases was even more haphazard. Modern experience shows that without treatment, cholera kills 40-60 per cent of its victims. As nineteenth-century Britain was without any effective treatment, this ratio may be used to infer the number of cases from the number of deaths and to detect exaggerated case figures in local accounts.

The demographic impact of cholera was small but significant. In the period 1838-68 in England and Wales the Registrar-General's figures show the cholera years as peaks in the mortality figures (Table 2). These figures must be put in perspective. The impact of cholera in 1849 only just exceeds that of the typhus which was brought to Britain in 1847 by refugees from the Irish famine, and, over a five-year period around 1849, deaths from common diarrhoea exceed deaths from cholera. In 1854, the two totals are nearly equal.

Although cholera was often compared to plague, the death rate was nothing like that of the medieval and seventeenth-century plagues. Historians have traditionally claimed that the 'Black Death' of 1349 killed between a third and a half of the population. In London the Bills of Mortality suggest that the later plagues killed between 15 and 25 per cent of the population.[2] The London cholera totals for 1849, 0.62 per cent, and for 1854, 0.43 per cent were minute beside the plague totals. Even the disaster villages of the cholera era did not approach the plague death rates. Newburn in County Durham lost 10 per cent of its

Prologue 13

Table 1: Cholera Deaths in Britain, 1831-1866

	England and Wales		Scotland	
Year	Cholera Deaths	Deaths per 1,000,000	Cholera Deaths	Deaths per 1,000,000
1831 1832	21,882[a]	–	9,592[a]	–
1848	1,908[b]	110[b]	6,000 to 7,000[c]	–
1849	53,293[b]	3,034[b]		
1853	4,419[b]	244[b]	6,848[d]	–
1854	20,097[b]	1,094[b]		
1866	14,378[b]	685[b]	1,270[e]	420[e]

Sources:
a. Derived from figures collected by Charles Creighton, *A History of Epidemics*, vol.2, p.816, 2nd edition, D.E.C. Eversley, E.A. Underwood and L. Overall (eds.), London, 1965. Creighton's figures seem more complete than those published by the Statistical Society or the 1849 Board of Health.
b. *Report on the cholera epidemic of 1866 in England,* supplement to the *29th Annual Report of the Registrar-General for Births, Deaths and Marriages for England and Wales,* P.P.,1867-8, vol.37.
c. Estimate from Board of Health returns in *Report of the General Board of Health on the epidemic of cholera in 1848 and 1849,* P.P.,1850, vol.21.
d. *16th Annual Report of the Registrar-General in England and Wales, Abstracts for 1854.* The total for Scotland was derived from the Board of Health returns, 31 August 1853 to 17 November 1854.
e. *12th detailed Annual Report of the Registrar-General of Births, Deaths and Marriages in Scotland,* P.P.,1868-9, vol.16.

Table 2: Crude Death Rate in England and Wales, 1846-56 and 1865-67

Year	Total Deaths	per 1,000	Year	Total Deaths	per 1,000
1846	390,315	23.06	1854	437,905	23.52*
1847	423,304	24.71	1855	425,703	22.61
1848	399,833	23.06	1856	390,506	20.51
1849	440,839	25.12*	....	....	....
1850	368,995	20.77	....	....	....
1851	395,396	21.99	1865	490,909	23.39
1852	407,135	22.38	1866	500,689	23.61*
1853	421,097	22.88	1867	471,073	21.98

*cholera years

Source: *31st Annual Report of the Registrar-General in England and Wales,* London, 1870.

population of 350, whilst at Bilston, where events horrified a country already suffering, 693 people died, 4.8 per cent of the total population of 14,492. None of these totals compare with the plague village of Eyam in Derbyshire where 259 died in a population of 350 during 1665-6.

Although the cholera epidemics of the nineteenth century can in no way be called demographic crises, the approach and arrival of these epidemics, especially that of 1832, created a crisis atmosphere in the country quite unlike that produced by any other threat apart from foreign invasion. The normally calm *Quarterly Review* viewed the approach of 'one of the most terrible pestilences which have ever desolated the earth' with considerable horror. It had killed fifty million people in fourteen years, the *Review* claimed, and threatened economic and social chaos as well as pain and death: 'If this malady should really take root and spread in these islands, it is impossible to calculate the horror even of its probable financial results alone.'[3] Cholera was a shock disease. It demanded and got attention from everyone, from all shades and all forms of opinion. This is its value for the historian. There are few other events or aspects of social life in early nineteenth-century Britain on which comments came from so many different places. There was a characteristic response from the religious periodicals and medical journals, from the radical newspapers and from magazines on household management; from the educational and temperance Press, and the literary and scientific papers. They all made some 'survey' of the literature and provided 'advice' for readers. The steady reporting of cases and deaths in the newspapers had the depressing effect of the tolling of a funeral bell. Many diseases killed more widely and killed more people than cholera, but few had such concentrated attention from so many. As the correspondent of the *Edinburgh Courant* commented on the border town of Jedburgh in 1849, 'The smallpox is still raging amongst us, numbering even more victims than the cholera; being as it were indigenous to the country, the dread of it is absorbed in the all pervading thought of cholera.'

There are many distinctive qualities about cholera that make an enquiry into the death of William Sproat more than an enquiry into the first of 140,000 dead. The question who or what killed William Sproat requires not only a medical answer but a close study of the workings of British society and its ability to defend itself. The immediate answer to the question may, with present-day medical knowledge, be given very simply. The keelman died from the effects of a micro-organism, the *cholera vibrio* which established itself in his intestines. Neither his doctors nor anyone else fully understood this until 1883, when the German researcher Koch identified the bacillus after several years' work in India and Egypt.[4]

The *cholera vibrio* invariably entered the human body by way of the mouth. Usually the potential victim swallowed water which had been infected by the excreta of another cholera sufferer. Cholera can also spread on infected food. The *vibrio* can survive two to five days in meat, milk and cheese and slightly less in green vegetables. Several fruits are especially favourable for cholera. In apples the *vibrio* can live for up to 16 days. It is worth remembering in light of much British reaction that cholera will last only eight hours in beer and wine. Although infected water supplies are the main means of spreading cholera, flies, infected clothing and blankets are also important. They transfer the *vibrio* to hands and food and so into the mouth and stomach. To develop successfully the *vibrio* must pass through the hostile acid environment of the stomach to the alkaline of the intestines. This need gives cholera the first of its important social characteristics. It is extremely difficult to develop the disease. Healthy individuals can survive quite heavy doses of infection. Macnamara recorded that out of 19 people drinking from an infected water vessel in 1876, only five contracted the infection. Normally the stomach acids, even the mild acidity of the saliva, will kill the *cholera vibrio*. But if the disease is difficult to contract, it is equally difficult to survive once the attack begins. Cholera kills by dehydration and kills rapidly, usually in three or four days, sometimes in a few hours. Once the *vibrio* is established, the victim develops the violent and characteristic symptoms so familiar to the doctors of 1832. Even without specific treatment the 50 per cent death rate declines towards the end of an epidemic visitation to any particular place. It is also lower in initially healthy people.

The symptoms of cholera develop in three stages, although nineteenth-century practice added a fourth, 'premonitory diarrhoea'. This arose from the belief that other bowel disorders, if allowed to develop, would become *cholera morbus*. This stage was associated with vague symptoms that were probably the beginning of the first stage of cholera proper. The patient appeared listless and depressed, and felt a little deaf though not unwell. He had 'indescribable sensations of being out of order' and 'perhaps an uncomfortable sensation of heat in the pit of the stomach'. As the *cholera vibrio* developed it embedded itself in the wall of the intestine, resulting in the reaction which shocked all who witnessed cholera cases. Violent vomiting and diarrhoea caused a massive loss of body fluids. This stage finished with the thin 'rice water' evacuations which contained part of the damaged lining of the intestine. As a result of this huge loss of fluid and possibly other chemical changes in the body, the patient suffered agonising muscular cramps. The dehydration did widespread damage to many organs of the body, especially the circulatory system. In the collapse stage which followed, pulse and temperature dropped and the excretion of all bodily fluids ceased. In the words of Edinburgh surgeon George Bell, who set out his experience in India for the benefit of his European colleagues,

> The eyes surrounded by a dark circle are completely sunk in the sockets, the whole countenance is collapsed, the skin is livid...The surface [of the skin] is now generally covered with cold sweat, the nails are blue, and the skin of the hands and feet are corrugated as if they had been long steeped in water...The voice is hollow and unnatural. If the case be accompanied by spasms, the suffering of the patient is much aggravated, and is sometimes excruciating...[5]

If the patient was fortunate and strong enough to survive this collapse stage, the stage at which most deaths occurred, he still had to face the consequent fever, which was part of the reaction and recovery phase and needed careful nursing. There were rare cases in which apparently healthy people dropped and died in a few moments in the street. These were widely reported and added to the terror of the disease. As the Methodists said,

> To see a number of our fellow creatures, in a good state of health, in the full possession of their wonted strength, and in the midst of their years, suddenly seized with the most violent spasms, and in a few hours cast into the tomb, is calculated to shake the firmest nerves, and to inspire dread in the stoutest heart.[6]

The symptoms were one source of terror. The unpredictable progress of the disease was another.[7] Cholera could creep slowly across country, missing whole towns and suburbs. Personal contact, food, clothes, a cloud of flies would drive it forward. Every so often a water supply would become infected and this relentless progress would be punctuated by an 'explosive' outbreak. Perhaps the excreta of a passing vagrant infected a stream, or the privy midden of a cholera family seeped into surrounding wells. When this happened cases appeared dozens at a time. Such outbreaks, like Gateshead, Newburn and Bilston were widely

Prologue

reported, adding to the terrifying reputation of cholera.

Cholera demands the historian's attention not just as the cause of public health reform or as an element of class tension, though it had some claim to be both, not just as evidence highlighting the insanitary conditions of industrial Britain, but as a test and a challenge. It was seen as a threat. The response to cholera tested many aspects of the working and quality of British society.

It tested the British understanding of natural events. Science, especially medicine and statistics, even the skills of theology and morals, were turned endlessly on the problem – all produced a chaos of ill-sorted fact and theories supported more by assertion than evidence. Cholera was a test of technology and resources. Once the skills of the water and sewage engineer had been developed it was possible to limit cholera, providing resources were made available to use these skills. Each epidemic was a test of administrative skills. The challenge needed a rapid and convincing response. Crucial decisions about quarantine and public health had to be taken with inadequate evidence. Men and medical supplies had to be found and distributed where needed. Above all, relevant information had to be collected and distributed to help individuals make their own plans. Cholera was a deep test of the values of British society, of the care which society felt it 'ought' to provide for those threatened, and the resources which it 'was' in fact prepared to provide. Because of the tension which cholera produced by its savagery and unpredictable movement, its approach and arrival was a severe test of social cohesion. To follow the cholera track was not just, as some observers claimed, to follow the track of filth and poverty, it was to watch the trust and co-operation between different parts of society strained to the utmost, especially the symbiotic tension of class relationships. Did British society have the social cohesion and stability to face the cholera? If so, what were the relationships, the institutions, the means of social control by which such stability was maintained?

The 1832 epidemic merits particular attention. Because it was first, comment and reaction were more widespread than in the later epidemics. Because it was the earliest of the epidemics, the contrast between our own patterns of thought and those of the nineteenth century are sharpest in 1832. The people of 1832 seem very close to the twentieth century in their behaviour. Their economic ambitions, their technology, their political ideas and social ambitions, even their dress is beginning to seem familiar, but the cholera revealed patterns of thought and reaction, especially in matters of medicine and religion, which were centuries away from our own.

The historian as ever is blessed with the gift of hindsight. He must judge the people of 1832 in light of an understanding of cholera which any reader could gain in half an hour from the local public library. He must find why a community of active, skilled and intelligent men failed to answer the question, 'what caused cholera and how can we stop it?' But judgement must be made at a second level. The enquiry is limited if all the efforts of 1832 are rejected as useless because they lacked the medical and scientific knowledge which was to come later; if the measures taken are only seen as the prehistory of our own 'successful' answer to the problem. The men of 1832 must be judged on their own terms: their administration judged as if whitewash and quarantine would stop cholera; their churchmen according to their views on the efficacy of prayer.

A number of studies of community reaction to disaster were made in the USA during the 1950s and 1960s.[8] The main interest was in the possible reaction of society to nuclear attack. Regularities of behaviour in communities struck by earthquake, flood, explosion or mass air attack were carefully observed. Panic was rare, but the response these communities made to the shock or threat of disruption often revealed more of their working and values than a study of a normal situation could have done. The processes which normally allocated resources and maintained stability were seen reacting rapidly to a new situation. Individuals and groups revealed much about their scale of values because they had to make rapid choices between social claims which in normal times would never come into conflict. Most studies revealed the prime claim which family had over work, friends and entertainment. Cholera was a creeping disaster so reaction was a little more studied and circumspect than reactions to a sudden impact disaster, but the manner in which it demanded attention and comment gave cholera the ability to reveal values, patterns of thought, patterns of social relationships and ways of allocating resources in the same way as a more sudden crisis.

The reactions of groups and individuals were influenced by their available resources and experience as well as by their values and expectations. Each situation tended to find the population divided into two groups, those with power and resources and those without. Those with power were expected to take action against cholera. Those without power were the likely victims. Each had a choice of action, quarantine, cleansing, medical provision, prayer or just doing nothing on the one hand, and flight, anger, alarm, obedience to regulations, or just doing nothing on the other. Values emerged in choices between life and

Prologue

property, between work and safety, between charitable action and government agencies. The resources of each group included material wealth, the value of their labour in the market, their social authority and prestige, their administrative and scientific skills and their technical ability. All these choices were influenced by the expectations which each group had of others, wage-earners of the medical profession, or of the local authority, and the administrator's expectations of reactions to the circular he was drafting. These expectations were all based on past experience of the physical as well as social world.

Because of the attention which it demanded, the terror it evoked, because of its unpredictable nature and because we now know that it was relatively simple to stop, cholera was well qualified to reveal the morbid pathology of British society in 1832.

Notes

1. W. Reid Clanny, *Hyperanthraxis, or the cholera in Sunderland,* London, 1832, pp.15-30; James Butler Kell, *The appearance of cholera at Sunderland in 1831,* Edinburgh, 1834, pp.22-34.
2. I. Sutherland, 'When was the great plague? Mortality in London, 1563-1665', in D.V. Glass and R. Revelle (eds.), *Population and Social Change,* London, 1972, pp.287-322; J.F.D. Shrewsbury, *Bubonic Plague in the British Isles,* Cambridge, 1970, pp.123 and 487, and the important review of this book by Christopher Morris in *Historical Journal,* vol.14, 1971, pp.205-34; Charles Creighton, *History of Epidemics in Britain,* 2nd edition, D.E.G. Eversley, E.A. Underwood and L. Overnall (eds.), London, 1965, pp.682 and 824; David Craigie, 'An account of the epidemic cholera at Newburn...', *Edinburgh Medical and Surgical Journal,* vol.37, 1832, p.337; Rev. W. Leigh, *An Authentic Narrative of the Melancholy Occurences at Bilston during the Awful Visitation in that Town of Cholera...,* Wolverhampton, 1833, states that 743 died in Bilston.
3. *Quarterly Review,* vol.46, 1832, p.170.
4. N.C. Macnamara, *Asiatic Cholera,* London, 1892.
5. George Hamilton Bell, *Treatis on the Cholera Asphyxia,* Edinburgh, 1831; the general account of cholera is taken from R. Pollitzer, *Cholera,* World Health Organisation, Geneva, 1959.
6. *Fraser's Magazine,* vol.4, 1831, p.613; *Methodist Magazine,* 1832, p.449.
7. *United Services Journal,* 1832, Part 3, p.449; Pollitzer, *Cholera,* p.733.
8. George W. Baker and Dwight D. Chapman (eds.), *Man and Society in Disaster,* New York, 1962.

2 APPROACH

In the winter of 1818-19, as the East India mails came in, the British Press began to take notice of a terrifying epidemic raging in Calcutta and the surrounding countryside. This 'new' disease, *cholera morbus*, had begun in Jessore in August 1817, and had already killed some 3,000 men out of the 10,000 strong army led by the Marquis of Hastings against the remains of the Marathi confederacy. There was nothing new about the disease in 1817 except the notice it gained from the British, who were then consolidating their power in India. Cholera had affected Calcutta in 1781-2 and two years later killed 20,000 pilgrims at Hurdwar, the great holy place of north India.[1] But in 1817 cholera changed its normal pattern of behaviour. It spread more rapidly than before, reached China, Persia and the Middle East, and in 1823 reached the Russian city of Astrakhan, where it halted. There may have been some mutation of the *cholera vibrio* which enabled it to spread with greater speed and savagery, but more likely the cause was some change in the economic and social conditions of India. The crucial period, 1810-30, saw no increase in the density of population, or the pace of internal migration, which might increase the spread of infection. If anything, war had reduced population in those years. Nor was there any improvement in internal transport, or any increase in internal trade, except in the port areas. Two changes did occur, both related to British influence in India and both related to the spread of cholera. Overseas trade had expanded, and this may have helped cholera spread into Persia, the vital land bridge with Europe. Within India the greatest change was in the nature of troop movements. The British now dominated large areas in all the major regions of India, and had instituted regular troop movements over the whole sub-continent. The rapid movement of units affected by cholera, like the army of the Marquis of Hastings, and the annual relief of troops on an all-India basis, which began in 1817, all broke down the regional barriers which had slowed the spread of epidemic.[2] By increasing the pace of war and trade in India, the European nations had stirred up a great well of infection in the swamps of Bengal, and so generated the four great pandemics which swept west in the nineteenth century.

Reaction to cholera in India was important for several reasons, and was part of the experience on which Britain drew in the summer of

1831. The initial reaction was one of total bewilderment and horror. Many years later one London physician remembered his feelings on being alone with a regiment, scant medical experience and cholera.

> Upon myself as the medical officer in charge the entire responsibility rested. To a young man of twenty five, what a fearful responsibility was the charge of a European regiment, with 2,000 native camp followers, and the cholera raging among them...coming as an epidemic never before in my life had I seen anything so awful as this disorder.[3]

This mixture of responsibility and helplessness was felt many times by medical men and administrators before the nineteenth century was done. There was a flurry of public health activity by the various provincial governments of India; early medical treatment was provided and a crop of rice banned in Bengal.[4] The three presidencies reacted to their failure to find an effective response to cholera by publishing a report each. These reports were the first substantial contribution to British medical knowledge of cholera. They were joined within a few years by several books written by medical men with Indian experience.

In a country where an adequate population census was not made until 1881 all statistical summaries of the impact of this first epidemic must be guesswork. M Moreau de Jonnes, a Frenchman from the Académie des Sciences with a breathtaking ability for making confident statistics from very little evidence, claimed that the first epidemic, by which he appears to mean the period 1817-23, attacked a tenth of the population and killed about a sixth of these. His case/death ratio was an unlikely one for cholera. His estimates may have been made from army figures which have a similar ratio and probably included a variety of bowel complaints. Between 1818 and 1822, 19,494 members of an army of 83,366 were attacked. In the five years, 23 per cent were attacked and 5 per cent died. The situation improved later in the decade, for the Bengal command reported losing 1.1 per cent of their men to cholera in the years 1826-32, whilst the overall death rate from all causes was 5.7 per cent.[5]

In 1826, cholera again began to spread rapidly. This time the trigger was the traditional one, the great Kumb festival at Hurdwar. Pilgrims from Lower Bengal brought cholera with them. They shared the water of the Ganges and the open crowded camps on its banks with pilgrims from other parts of India, who then carried cholera back to their homes. Cholera spread along the trade routes to Tehran, Baku and Astrakhan

Approach 23

and up the Volga. It was taken across the caravan routes of the Hindu Kush and the Kirghiz Steppe to reach Orenburg in August 1829. The military cordon which had worked in 1823 proved inadequate to stop this second epidemic. As the merchants from southern and European Russia gathered for the great autumn fair in Nijni-Novgorod, cholera appeared in the town. The merchants dispersed rapidly, further spreading the disease.[6] The appearance of cholera in Moscow in September 1830 was a clear warning to the rest of Europe. Moscow was a city with European standards of culture and civilisation. The British realised that cholera was no longer just a problem for the East India administration. 'If the scourge reached Moscow, nothing could prevent it spreading over Europe.'[7] Throughout 1831, cholera drove its way across northern Europe with the help of a savage military campaign in Poland, and the incessant coming and going along the interlocking trade routes of a commercial continent in search of profit. The Russian advance on the army of their rebellious Polish subjects and the chaos caused by Polish refugees drove cholera west with greater speed. A Prussian military cordon was brushed aside with ease. A similar cordon around St Petersburg only caused a slight delay in the spread of the disease. By mid summer cholera was in the Baltic flax port of Riga where that year's crop was arriving for export to Britain. By October it had reached Hamburg, only a few hours sailing time from the east coast of England. Together they were a major threat to Britain.[8]

The responsibility for responding to this threat lay initially with the Privy Council. By 1831, the Privy Council had become the odd job man of the constitution. It dealt with friendly societies, French *émigrés* and Catholic oaths, as well as quarantine; it had spawned the active and growing Board of Trade, and was to be the base from which the departments of Health and Education were to emerge.[9] Because its organisation was so vague and political control weak, the civil servants at the Privy Council had more power and independence than most. Charles Greville, in whose diaries cholera mingles with many other political concerns, was the Clerk to the Council and was directed to superintend quarantine stations.[10] His immediate adviser was Sir William Pym, Superintendent-General of Quarantine, a military surgeon whose experience qualified him for the job as well as anyone in Britain. During his naval service he had directed medical operations against several outbreaks of plague and yellow fever, which until 1831 were the major diseases which concerned the quarantine authorities.

The quarantine regulations of 1831 were a development of the eighteenth-century fight to exclude plague and keep out yellow fever. Basic tactics were still those outlined in the regulations devised by Dr Richard Mead during the plague threat of 1720. Since the 1700s ships from plague areas had to do 40 days quarantine with a foul bill of health and 21 days with a clean bill, mostly at the main quarantine station in Standgate Creek on the Medway. Attempts to build a lazaretto at nearby Chetney Hill in the 1800s failed to materialise. During the French wars these regulations, which included the death penalty among their sanctions, were increasingly attacked by commercial interests. Liverpool merchants found the delays to Levant cotton an expensive inconvenience, even when they had their own quarantine station at Milford Haven. The Levant Company, by then a merchant pressure group in London, hired a physician called MacLean who confidently told Parliament that plague was not infectious, despite having caught the disease himself on a trip to Constantinople. After two Select Committees, a milder and more flexible statute was passed in 1825. Its regulations were backed by fines of up to £400, and Pym was appointed to work the Act, which he did with every effort to limit the delays to commercial life without ignoring the risks of infection.[11]

When the Privy Council learned that cholera was in Riga, and 700 to 800 ships loaded with flax and hemp were ready to sail for Britain, quarantine under the 1825 Act was declared for all ships from Russia, the Baltic, the Cattegat and the Elbe. This was extended to other west European ports when cholera reached Hamburg. Such ships were to proceed to a series of quarantine stations ranging from Milford Haven to Cromarty Bay, including Standgate. There was a quiet, almost desperate realisation that effective quarantine was Britain's only real hope of escape. The appeal for strict observance was made, not so much because of the penalties but, 'upon serious consideration of the great extent of misery and calamity which a single instance of improvidently neglecting any of these regulations may bring upon our loving subjects'. In 1831, Standgate handled 3,080 ships instead of the usual two or three hundred.[12] It operated effectively and there were no cholera scares and rumours in the Thames and approaches that summer to hint that infected men and goods were being let ashore. But for the customs officers controlling the smaller quarantine stations, the increase of work was more than they could effectively police and cholera broke the net.

As soon as the British realised the threat which was moving across Europe, there was a desperate search for authentic information about a disease which seemed more terrible because its nature was unknown and its working ill-understood. Greville began his job by writing to a British

Approach 25

physician in Moscow asking for information. Dr Walker explained what he could and was written off by Greville as 'a very useless and inefficient agent', but the published parts of Walker's letters show that he only shared the general bewilderment caused by cholera. He confirmed that Russia had the same disease as India; even this had been in doubt at the start of the year. He noted that half the patients died, but could not be sure of its infectious nature. Yes, it moved along the lines of water communication, the boatmen were often first to suffer, but then many contacts, especially in hospitals, failed to get the cholera. Yes, the Russians had a 14-day quarantine between Moscow and St Petersburg, but many of their medical profession thought the disease was not contagious. Such doubts could hardly delight Greville, who had just brought an important section of British commerce to a halt, and needed more than a few vague letters to defend his conduct.[13]

He also needed authoritative advice to quiet increasing public alarm. On 9 June, he consulted Sir Henry Halford, President of the Royal College of Physicians, sending him all the papers on cholera which the government had received. Halford stated that cholera was infectious and needed 14 days quarantine. The Royal College, somewhat jealous of its President's solo performance, insisted on giving its collective opinion and concluded that cholera was not only infectious but could be carried by cloth, raw flax or wool. Halford and Greville decided that a medical mission to St Petersburg was the only way to improve their knowledge and chose Dr William Russell and Dr David Barry for the task. Barry already had government experience, reporting on the Gibraltar yellow fever in 1828. On 18 June Greville asked Halford for names of members of the College to serve on a Central Board of Health which was to advise the Privy Council on the best defences against cholera. This followed the precedent of 1805 when a similar board had been set up to advise on measures against the yellow fever then in Gibraltar. The request for an opinion from the Royal College followed the example of 1824 when cholera had been in eastern Europe.[14] The government's first response consisted of two moves from the pigeon holes of the past.

On 21 June the names of the Central Board were published in the *London Gazette*. It read like a roll-call from the London bedsides of Court, aristocracy and wealth. In the chair was Sir Henry Halford, President of the College. The *Lancet* might sneer at him as a courtier of the Vaughan connection, but this was a formidable family alliance, the very mixture of success and influence which bound the élite of the old professions to the ruling classes of Britain. From the nine sons of a Leicester physician there came Sir Henry, a Judge of Common Pleas who was also a Privy Councillor, the Dean of Chester, Warden of Merton College Oxford, and an Envoy to the United States, again on the Privy Council. An Oxford education, pleasing manners and a marriage into the aristocracy had brought Sir Henry the leading London practice of the late twenties. He included four sovereigns among his patients. Henry Holland was as well known for his travels in the eastern Mediterranean as for his extensive practice in London society. Dr William George Maton had made the acquaintance of the King and Queen at Weymouth through his interest in botany. He attended the Duke of Kent and went on to share the best London practice with Halford. Dr Thomas Turner was Treasurer of the College. Pelham Warner had another large London practice despite his cold manner and reputation as a huge snuff-taker. William MacMichael was another Court physician and friend of Halford's. During the summer of 1831 he wrote an incisive summary of current knowledge to justify the Board's quarantine policy. Last came James Edward Seymour, brought in as secretary to the Board.[15] The rest were civil servants, Sir T. Byam, Comptroller of the Navy, Edward Stewart, deputy chairman from the Customs Board, Sir William Burnett, Commissioner from the Victualling Office, Sir James McGrigor, another fellow of the College, a man with extensive service experience in India, the West Indies and Europe and now Director-General of Army Hospitals, and finally Sir William Pym.

When this board fell from prominence in November, the *Lancet*, never a friend of the Royal College, dismissed them as a crowd of drones, sycophants and courtiers, who had never had any personal experience of treating cholera.[16] They were certainly courtiers, and there was little evidence that any of them had ever treated cholera, though several had seen the other quarantine fevers. By attacking the Board of Health on the grounds that its members knew nothing of cholera, the *Lancet* was very deliberately missing the point. The government needed authority for their actions. The *Lancet* believed that authority should rest upon rigorous practical training and knowledge, upon science-based research and upon the medical man's ability as a practitioner. The government sought that mixture of social prestige, birth and connection, and real ability which contributed to a man's social status in the aristocratic commercial society which had evolved over the eighteenth century. The Royal College was the élite body of the medical profession, men usually from wealthy middle-class families well groomed by the aristocratic classical education of Oxford and Cambridge. The seven men on the Board were the élite of the élite. It mattered not that they had never seen cholera. They could, and did ask those who had. What mattered was that they shared the authority of the ruling class, and authority was needed for decisions of government. The ruling class consulted these men on medically based matters of state just as they would consult them about their own health. A man who could advise on the health of the King could surely advise on the health of the nation.

Feelings in the country polarised into the alarmed and the apathetic. Both were products of uncertainty. Many felt vague apprehension. Even Southey in the remote safety of Keswick wrote, 'I wake in the morning with a sense of insecurity', and by October alarm and agitation were evident in the House of Commons. 'Did the government realise Hamburg was only 36 hours steaming time away from Britain?' asked Sir Richard Vyvyan. It was a mistake to think that crossing the sea would reduce the virulence of cholera. No precaution was too much, said Warburton. There was alarm in Northumberland, said another MP, and even the cynical and relaxed radical, Hume, pressed for more government action.[17] After the epidemic the short-lived radical journal *Carpenter's Political Magazine*, though mainly interested in parliamentary reform, enquired:

> into the sources of those alarming accounts which have been officially, and at the same time so assiduously, circulated throughout the land, as not only to dismay the timid, and perplex and astonish the ignorant, but even for a time to confound the minds of the well informed,[18]

and blamed the public Press. The riots in St Petersburg and Moscow, the deaths in the military camps of Poland, and colourful accounts of disaster in distant Asiatic cities did little more than feed idle curiosity for news and perhaps a Gothic taste for horror, but when cholera was a few days or hours away, such reports were the basis for all manner of fears. One of the Scottish Missionary Papers described the social chaos in Astrakhan: 'business of every kind was at a stand, the bank suspended its operations; in the bazaar not a whisper was to be heard; even the cabaks (tippling houses) were abandoned.'[19] Others produced a series of formidable cholera death totals from across the world: Mauritius, 20,000, Java, 102,000, a quarter of the population of Orenburg, and laced the diet with details of the plague. The nature of the newspaper and periodical Press as a media is, and was, to select striking details to gain and retain the interest of readers. This, as always, increased the apparent tension, violence and pace of an incident. The very language of the articles was calculated to increase alarm — scourge, plague, pestilence, Asiatic violence, devastation, rampage, desperate, formidable, capricious, mysterious, intractable and so on. It was a diet which promised social and economic confusion to a waiting country. Others, like *John Bull* and the *Asiatic Magazine,* deliberately said nothing on the grounds that this would reduce alarm. Another group, amongst them many medical men, assured the public that when cholera came it would not be as bad in Britain as elsewhere. The varied climate, prosperity, 'our insular position', 'the modern habits of our people', 'superior clothing, comfort and diet', and 'the easier condition of the lower orders', were all suggested as factors which would protect Britain from the full force of the epidemic.[20] The more thoughtful, like the *Monthly Review,* a very ordinary literary review for the middle-class drawing room, suggested taking action on diet, cleanliness and ventilation, rather than 'filling our minds with chimerical horrors'.[21]

During the summer of 1831, the government became convinced that their decision on quarantine had been correct. The decision rested on the debate between the contagionist and non-contagionist (or miasmatic) schools of thought concerning the etiology of cholera. Contagionists, like the Royal College of Physicians, claimed that cholera was 'communicable from person to person', whilst their opponents believed that the disease spread without any contact with existing cases, and was caused by changes in the atmosphere, vapour from the earth or rotting vegetation.[22]

The evidence available to the government in the summer of 1831 was inconclusive. Here lay the strength of the anti-quarantine lobby. At first it might have seemed self-evident that cholera was contagious. Two out of three of the early Indian Government reports of 1819-20 said so, as did all the official Russian Government papers, including the 1830 report of the Medical Council of St Petersburg, which was summarised for the British Parliament in 1831. It followed the roads and major trade routes; the first victims were often travellers; the boatmen had been first to suffer along the Volga, and when rigid quarantine was enforced isolated places had been able to escape. A double cordon of troops had sealed off Zarcozelo and Peterhoff and prevented the cholera of nearby Moscow reaching the court, nobility and their attendants. The letters which the Privy Council began to get from Russell and Barry in July only served to confirm this view.[23]

Closer examination of the evidence quickly brought doubts. The contagionist Board of Health must have listened with dismay to the Indian medical men they interviewed in July. Of the seven men whose evidence survives, four were anti-contagionist and three were undecided. Dr Daun, surgeon of the 89th Regiment, and Mr Wybrow, surgeon to the 17th Lancers, both found the evidence conflicting. Dr Alexander from the Bombay area rejected contagion on the grounds that the hospital attendants had escaped. In their published works other Indian men tended to be equally against contagion. Even the Russians were beginning to admit that cholera was less infectious than plague and that their quarantine nets were less than effective.[24] Despite such doubts the Board maintained the correctness of quarantine, even when they were replaced in November.

The Privy Council declared a 14-day quarantine under the 1825 Act. When the Royal College of Physicians decided that cholera could be carried by rags, cordage and cloth, the Central Board of Health devised a complex series of rules for airing and drying goods, which applied especially to the flax and hemp ships coming from the Baltic.[25] The commercial interests trading with the Baltic were naturally the first to complain. Over 3,000 ships were delayed an expensive 14 days in government quarantine stations, where they paid a government fee of £5.14s.6d., as well as extra wages for captain and crew. The London merchants claimed that the delay meant that ships could only make one trip in the 1831 season instead of the usual two, thus adding further to losses. Greville was irritated by the alarm of 'Scotch merchants for their cargoes', but found Poullett-Thompson, President of the Board of Trade, himself a merchant, 'disgusted' by the June regulations. *John Bull,* always suspicious of Whig government, claimed that Poullett-Thompson was responsible for not stopping the Baltic trade earlier in the year, but there was no evidence that he had influenced the decision at all.[26]

The quarantine did have a marginal influence on the flax trade. The official values of imported raw materials for the textile industry show that whilst imports of raw wool and cotton increased between 1830 and 1831, the import of flax dropped. The flax figures were between 5 and 10 per cent below what might have been expected if they had followed the same trend as wool and cotton. The following year flax imports increased whilst the others fell, suggesting that manufacturers were making up stocks which had been depleted by the difficulties of 1831. During 1832 wool imports suffered from very tough quarantine regulations imposed by the Spaniards who supplied an important part of the British woollen industry.[27]

It would be wrong to suggest that the whole of the British manufacturing interest was waiting for a chance to discredit quarantine. One Leeds wool merchant warned the Central Board of the danger of bales of wool being unpacked in crowded factories after they had come from Germany. In July, John Marshall, millionaire leader of the West Riding flax industry, wrote to the Board, warning them that a large import of flax was due:

> you may know that we are engaged in the superintendence of a manufactory, I may just explain that we use a great deal of flax, the produce of Lithuania...which is shipped from the port of Kiev and we are therefore most anxious to do all in our power to prevent the spread of the disease in our country even after the flax has undergone all the precautions of strict quarantine. If the disease be infectious and that infection can be conveyed through the intervention of materials or goods, there can be no material more capable of conveying it than flax, every pound of which has been half or three quarters of an hour in the hands of a peasant during the operation of swinging when he must frequently have been in a state of perspiration...[28]

The attack on quarantine began cautiously. Public opinion in the summer of 1831 made any relaxation of the regulations impossible. The radical MP, Joseph Hume, whose demands gained extra authority because he sat for the huge constituency of Middlesex, took the opportunity to press for the abolition of the quarantine fees, and was joined by Alderman Thompson, speaking for the London shipping interests, and Matthew White Ridley for the commercial powers of Newcastle and the north-east. Poulett-Thompson replied that the government planned to abolish the fees on 1 January 1832 and would not change that date.[29] As the failure of quarantine became evident, commercial interests made more direct attacks on the regulations. Quarantine was blamed for lay-offs in Manchester during December. Some of the east coast ports blamed their inability to raise money for anti-cholera measures on the loss of trade brought by the regulations.[30] The government were still prepared to defend their policy in public, claiming in January 1832 that it was the only effective way to stop cholera from entering Britain. It was an odd claim in view of the existence of cholera in the north, and the Central Board had already begun to express doubts. Quarantine, they warned, was not based upon any knowledge of the disease, but was 'kept up, partly from ill-defined apprehension and partly from reverence for old institutions'.[31] On 13 February, as soon as cholera had been confirmed in London, Hume and his allies renewed their attack. Cutting commercial contact, they claimed, made the evils of the disease worse by adding 'famine and destitution' to pestilence. A new note of

Approach

concern for the poor was added to concern for the freedom of trade: 'the best preventative [said Hume] was to provide the poor and destitute with wholesome food, and fuel, and raiment, and to enforce rigid habits of cleanliness'.[32] The government admitted the futility of the regulations now that cholera was established in London. In March, they were dropped.

The debate over contagion and miasma in the summer of 1831 was scientifically inconclusive but politically it was a victory for the contagionists. The first result of this victory was the quarantine policy which failed. The Board of Health anticipating the arrival of cholera considered the possibility of internal quarantine to limit its spread. This was rejected as impracticable and instead the policy of isolating first cases and separating the sick from the healthy was recommended. The policy and the measures recommended to accompany it needed a sophisticated local administration. For this reason, the Board advised on the creation of an extensive network of local boards of health. Although local boards and committees had acted in health matters before — there had been the Manchester Board which acted as a pressure group for factory regulation in the 1790s, and several committees which had pressed smallpox inoculation — nothing had ever been tried on this scale. The local board of health, an executive agency drawing on local sources of power and authority and loosely linked to a central agency, was one major innovation of the first cholera epidemic, and an innovation never to be repeated in that particular form. Such an extensive network was first envisaged by the Central Board of Health in July 1831, as they worked out the logic of the contagionist position in terms of positive action. The first job of the local board of health was early detection, which they felt could prevent a serious epidemic developing in any area. When a case was reported, the Central Board envisaged a hoard of 'expurgators' descending on the house with carts and conveyances. The sick would be removed to hospital, and if they recovered, to the convalescent house. All contacts would be put in an isolation house. The three buildings must be separate but might be put in the same enclosure so they could be easily guarded. The Board suggested the local military could do this job. The expurgators would then purify the house; rags, cordage and paper destroyed; for clothing and furniture, 'strong effusions' of water and boiling in strong leys; chloride of lime for drains and privies, and hot lime wash for the walls from garret to cellar and on top of all this the free admission of air for a week. The expurgators were to live apart from the public, and the dead to be buried in ground close to the house for the infected. The

Board felt that the 'violence done to ordinary feelings', even the splitting of families, would be worth while in order to stop cholera.[33] It was a wonderful, complete, logical scheme, but without a jot of human feeling or understanding.

In November 1831, the Privy Council made a sudden change in the form of the Central Board of Health. On 22 November, the *London Gazette* announced the names of a new Board: the Hon. Edward Stewart (chairman) and William Pym from the quarantine department, Lt.-Colonel John Marshall and Major R. MacDonald, half-pay officers who were to get £400 a year for their cholera work, Russell, late of the East India service, to get £730, and David Barry, another half-pay man £511, and William MacLean the secretary, £250 – Colonel Rowan from the police department was named but does not seem to have acted. The change was a logical one in the circumstances of November but seems to have been made with little regard for the professional and collegiate pride of the physicians. By November these men had done the job they were best qualified to do. They had lent their authority to steady the nerves of government in a period of public alarm. They had gathered an enormous amount of information and opinion on the etiology, nature and treatment of cholera. The government welcomed the élite of the Royal College as advisors, but as cholera began to spread in north-east England, the nature of the task changed. The Privy Council Office realised that the burden of day-to-day administration would increase, and must have shared the feelings of one MP who asked if the eminent members of the Board were not too busy with their own affairs to bother with cholera. The papers of the old Board were bundled up with scant ceremony and passed over to a team of administrators who could work full-time. They were men more familiar with office routine, with the mixture of tact and firmness needed to deal with local enquiries and local obstinacy. In Russell and Barry, the Board now included men who had seen and treated cholera in European conditions, men who realised the medical and social difficulties which this involved. The Board was chosen for its bureaucratic skills and medical experience, not its social status and authority.[34]

Other issues lay below the surface. The plans of the first Board included strong coercive measures for isolating first cases. The second Board rejected this and decided to rely on persuasion. Russell and Barry had both seen Russian methods of coercion result in riot and disorder, and anticipated that the British population would take even less kindly to such measures. Greville's diary showed that the Privy Council Office was becoming increasingly irritated with its strongly

Approach 33

contagionist Board of Health, especially the cumbersome regulations for treating goods and textiles.[35] Although the Council supported the Board until November, their first action after the change was to ask the physicians to lend their authority to a relaxation of regulations. They got a firm 'no change' answer from the ousted Board already offended by brusque treatment, and not until January did the new Board pluck up courage to reduce quarantine from 15 to 10 days.[36] The new Board was attacked by Halford because it lacked the confidence of the medical profession and by Hume because it lacked the confidence of the City of London (it contained no anti-contagionists), but public reception of the reports issued by these Boards showed that the November change was largely unnoticed.[37]

The results of the Board's work in the summer of 1831 were seen in three comprehensive circulars issued on 20 October, 14 November and 13 December 1831, which Dr Barry called their 'Pastorals'.[38] The rules and regulations of 20 October were published before the first Sunderland cases were known. It was hoped that quarantine would be successful. They began with a shrill plea for 'vigilance', and an especial warning against smugglers from Europe visiting the small fishing villages along the coast. The Board wanted all magistrates and clergy to make special appeals to the local population on the subject. The magistrates and the clergy were the traditional focus of authority in the localities and, in the absence of an administrative structure for the job in hand, the Central Board turned to them and other elements of the local élite for help:

> There should be established a local board of health, to consist of the Chief and other Magistrates, the Clergyman of the parish, two or more Physicians or Medical Practitioners, and three or more of the Principal Inhabitants...

The Board was ambivalent on the question of coercion. Internal quarantine was hinted at:

> All intercourse with any infected town, and the neighbouring country, must be prevented by the best means within the power of the Magistrates, who will make regulations for the supply of provisions...

The use of troops and police cordons was threatened in extreme cases. The immediate separation of the sick from the healthy' was thought to be the only way of stopping the spread of cholera. Those who refused to be removed to hospital were to be isolated in their own houses with the word 'sick' painted on the door. The cleansing measures were much the same as the July plan with special emphasis placed on burial in detached ground.

The magistrates and clergy were asked to mitigate the conditions in which cholera spread:

> the poor, ill-fed, and unhealthy part of the population, and especially those who have been addicted to the drinking of spirituous liquors, and indulgence in irregular habits, have been the greatest sufferers from the disease...

The disease had spread most rapidly in the dirty and crowded parts of the big towns. There followed a description of the symptoms from Russell and Barry – a crucial aid for doctors who had never seen the disease. The treatment they suggested was mainly for restoring the circulation by hot blankets, mustard and linseed poultices, and bags of hot salt and bran. The circular was printed in the *London Gazette* and appeared in several different mamphlet forms. Most newspapers printed the whole circular for their readers, and periodicals as varied as *Carpenter's Political Magazine* and the *Edinburgh Medical and Surgical Journal* reviewed the Board's work, in general, with a welcome and some comments of their own on cholera.[39]

Only the *Lancet* attacked the circular. They disliked the minor place which was given to the medical profession on the local boards. The *Lancet* represented the most radical claims of the general practitioner for professional recognition. Within the month the administrators had given equal offence to the most aristocratic element in the profession in their brush with Sir Henry Halford and the first Central Board of Health. This was early evidence of the tension between medical men and administrators which, under the tactless influence of Edwin Chadwick, was to bedevil British public health for half a century.

The second circular, of 14 November 1831, was based on the five months' study made by Russell and Barry in Europe. The local boards were to report to the Central Board. The policy of these boards was to be carried into effect by inspectors who would make house-to-house visitations in the districts into which the territory of each local board was divided. Deficiencies found by the inspectors were to be remedied 'by every means individual and public charitable exertion can supply'. Where this policy was followed a well-thought-out bureaucratic structure was created, but the local boards and the inspectors had few sanctions and slender authority. The Central Board was now clear. The members 'strongly depreciate all measures of coercion'. 'Good sense and good feeling' were relied upon to support quarantine and isolation. The public were warned that no specific treatment existed for cholera and were advised to avoid chill and loose bowels, and to pay attention to fresh air and cleanliness, though 'the true preventatives are a healthy body and a cheerful unruffled mind.'

The second circular was a distinct softening of the contagionist policies of the Central Board.

The document of 13 December extended many of the themes of November. More details were given of cleansing and burials, and the need for early information emphasised (still a contagion measure). Quarantine was not mentioned but the local community was urged to give special attention to the poor:

> It is of utmost importance to the public health that an improved diet, and flannel clothing, at least flannel belts and woollen stockings, should be given to the poor. No person should ever allow himself to sit down and get cool with wet feet. . . . The most effectual means by which this disease may be prevented from extending, is to enable the poor, who are generally the first attacked, to oppose to its influence, as far as practicable by those ameliorations in diet, clothing, and lodging which public and private charity, will it is hoped not fail to produce.

This suggestion was much nearer to miasmatist analysis for it was an effort to remove those predisposing causes which enabled 'the infected atmosphere' to attack the victim. The full practical effect of these circulars can only be seen in a study of the localities, but it is clear from this summary that the government, caught in the confusion of the contagion-miasma argument, faced two choices: contagion meant quarantine with loss of trade and disruption of family life – miasma meant cleansing and poor relief on a massive scale, expensive for rates and charitable subscriptions. The government, faced with two unpopular policies, and no pressing scientific justification for either, chose like many governments in the same position, to do a little bit of both and did neither very well.

Notes

1. *Times*, 14 October and 27 November 1818 and 2 February 1819; R. Pollitzer, *Cholera*, p.12; N.C. Macnamara, *History of the Asiatic Cholera from 1781 to July 1892*, London, 1892, p.7; figures from *Reports on the Epidemic Cholera, which has raged through Hindustan and the Peninsular of India, since August 1817*, published under the authority of the Government of Bombay, Bombay, 1819, reviewed by *Edinburgh Medical and Surgical Journal*, vol.16, 1820, p.458.
2. R.H. Kennedy, *Notes on the Epidemic Cholera*, Calcutta, 1827, pp.53 and 74, reviewed in *E.M.S.J.*, vol.28, 1827, p.427.
3. *Memorable Events in the Life of a London Physician*, London, 1863. The copy in the Edinburgh University Library attributes authorship to Dr Samuel Dickson.
4. *Asiatic Journal*, vol.5, 1818, p.447.
5. *E.M.S.J.*, vol.25, 1826, p.168, quoting James Annesley, *Sketches of the Most Prevalent Diseases of India. . .*, London, 1825; *E.M.S.J.*, vol.41, 1834, p.390.
6. A.C. Banerjea, 'Note on Cholera in the United Provinces (Uttar Pradesh),*Indian Journal of Medical Research*, vol.39, 1951; R. Pollitzer, *Cholera*, pp.21-3; David Craigie, 'Account of the Asiatic Cholera as it appeared in the confines of Europe and Asia and eventually proceeded to Moscow, translated from the German edition of the Official Reports of the Russian Government. . .', *E.M.S.J.*, vol.37, 1832, supplement, p.lvii.
7. *Eclectic Review*, 3rd series, vol.5, 1831, p.244; *London Medical and Physical Journal*, vol.66, 1831.
8. R. Pollitzer, *Cholera*, p.22; David Craigie, 'On the Progress of Cholera through the West of Russia to Poland, translated and abridged from German Reports', *E.M.S.J.*, vol.37, 1832, supplement, p.cxxxii; *United Services Journal*, 1831, Pt.II, pp.258 and 410.
9. Sir William Blackstone, *Commentaries on the Laws of England*, 4 vols., 17th edition, London, 1830, with notes and additions by Edward Christian, Esq.; M.S. Giuseppi, *Guide to the contents of the Public Record Office*, revised edition, HMSO, 1963, vol.II, p.233.
10. *The Greville Memoirs*, Henry Reeves (ed.), 8 vols., 1888, vol.II, p.59.
11. 'Contagion and Quarantine', *Quarterly Review*, vol.27, 1822, pp.524-53; 'Plague, a contagious disease', *Quarterly Review*, vol.33, 1826, pp.218-57; *S.C. Appointed to Consider the Validity of the Doctrine of Contagion in the Plague*, P.P., 1819, II; *Second Report of the S.C. Appointed to Consider Means of Improving the Foreign Trade of the Country: Quarantine*, P.P. (H. of C.), 1824, IV; *An Act to Repeal the Several Laws Relating to Quarantine, and to make other Provisions in Lieu thereof*, 6 George IV, c.78; Charles F. Mullet, 'A century of English Quarantine (1709-1825)', *Bulletin of the History of Medicine*, vol.23, 1949, pp.527-45; P. Froggatt, 'The Lazaret at Chetney Hill', *Medical History*, vol.8, 1964, pp.44-62.
12. *London Gazette*, 14 June 1831; Letter from Sir William Pym, 7 June 1831, printed in *Copies or Extracts of all information Communicated to His Majesty's Government Relative to the Cholera Morbus*, P.P. (H. of C.), 1831, XVIII; *A Return showing the number of vessels having performed Quarantine at Standgate Creek from 1st January 1826 to 1st January 1844*, P.P. (H. of Lords), 1844, XV.
13. *Copies. . .of all information. . .relative to Cholera; The Greville Memoirs*, vol.II, p.154.
14. *The Greville Memoirs*, pp.154, 158 and 222; *Times*, 16 June 1831.
15. William Munk, *The Life of Sir Henry Halford, bart.*, London, 1875; William Munk, *The Roll of the Royal College of Physicians*, 4 vols., London, 1878; William MacMichael, *Is the Cholera Spasmodica of India a contagious Disease. . .a*

letter addressed to Sir Henry Halford, London, 1831.
16. Fraser Brockington, 'Public Health at the Privy Council, 1831-34', *Journal of the History of Medicine*, April 1961, pp.161-85; The Earl of Oxford made a similar protest in the House of Lords but got little reaction from the government, *Hansard's Parliamentary Debates*, 3rd series, vol.4, col.357, House of Lords, 27 June 1831.
17. John Warter Wood (ed.), *Selections from the letters of Robert Southey*, 4 vols., London, 1836, vol.iv, p.225; L.J. Jennings (ed.), *The Correspondence and Diaries of Hon. John Wilson Croker, LL.D., F.R.S., Secretary of the Admiralty 1809-1830*, 3 vols., London, 1884, vol.ii, p.149; *Hansard's Parliamentary Debates*, 3rd series, vol.7, col. 898.
18. *Carpenter's Political Magazine*, Part II, 1831-2, p.48.
19. *Lancet*, 12 March 1831.
20. *Fraser's Magazine*, vol.4, 1831-2, pp.613-25; Bisset Hawkins, *History of the Epidemic Spasmodica Cholera*, London, 1831; *United Services Journal*, Part III, 1832, pp.449-58; *E.M.S.J.*, vol.36. 1831, p.118.
21. *The Monthly Review*, n.s., vol.II, 1831, pp.504-9.
22. *Copies or Extracts. . .relative to Cholera Morbus*, P.P. (H. of C.), 1831, vol.XVII; Eight relates the debate in more detail.
23. 'On the Malignant Cholera', *E.M.S.J.*, vol.37, 1832, p.203; 23 July 1831, P.R.O., P.C.1/101.
24. Evidence of the Medical Practitioners in India, P.R.O., P.C.1/106; this evidence was subsequently published along with the reports from Russia as *Official Reports made to the Government by Drs. Russell and Barry on the disease called Cholera Spasmodica. . .*, London, 1832, published by authority of H.M. Most Honourable Privy Council, copy in P.C.1/109; Fraser Brockington, art. cit.
25. *Copies or Extracts of all Information. . .relative to Cholera Morbus*, P.P. (H. of C.), 1831, XVII.
26. *John Bull*, 13 Nov. 1831.
27. B.R. Mitchell and P. Deane, *Abstract of British Historical Statistics*, Cambridge, 1962, pp.291-2.
28. 1 July 1831, P.R.O., P.C.1/101.
29. *Hansard's Parliamentary Debates*, 3rd series, vol.6, col.455, 23 August 1831.
30. *The Greville Memoirs*, 8 December 1831.
31. *Cholera Gazette*, no.1, 14 Jan. 1832; Document prepared by the Central Board of Health on the Communicability of Cholera, 4 January 1831, P.R.O., P.C.1/103.
32. *Hansard's Parliamentary Debates*, 3rd series, vol.10, 1832, col.268.
33. 11 July 1831, P.R.O., P.C.1/101.
34. Fraser Brockington, art. cit.
35. *The Greville Memoirs*, 8 July 1831.
36. William Munk, *The Life of Sir Henry Halford*, London, 1895; *Cholera Gazette*, no.1, 14 January 1832.
37. *Hansard's Parliamentary Debates*, 3rd series, vol.10, col.534, 20 February 1832.
38. Major Macdonald, Royal Hotel, Edinburgh, 28 December 1831, P.R.O., P.C.1/107.
39. *John Bull*, 31 Oct. 1831; *E.M.S.J.*, vol.36. 1831, p.404; *Carpenter's Political Magazine*, vol.1, December 1831.

3 SUNDERLAND

Whilst the implications of these circulars were being examined by administrators and public, the dark comedy of Sunderland was enacted on the north-east coast of England. Sunderland was the first place to experience cholera and hence attracted a great deal of attention in newspapers, pamphlets and histories. The day-to-day relationships, the fears of unemployment, the commercial greed and professional pride in the insecure prosperity of a major port gave cholera the perfect means to enter and spread throughout Britain.

Sunderland had prepared itself as conscientiously as any place in the kingdom. On 18 June 1831, during the first cholera scare occasioned by the gazetting of the Central Board of Health, Sunderland had formed a Board of Health. The chief magistrate was in the chair, but most of the work of the Board was done by its medical committee, which elected Dr Reid Clanny as chairman. He was the leader of the medical profession in the town, for he was senior physician at Sunderland General Infirmary. By 1830 most big towns had their general infirmary and several other hospitals, all supported by voluntary subscriptions; the senior medical posts, physicians and surgeons were all honorary, held by the leading practitioners in the town, elected by the subscribers. These posts were much prized by medical men. The reputation they brought assured the holder of an extensive practice among the wealthiest, highest fee-paying members of the local population. William Reid Clanny was an ex-naval surgeon who had qualified as a physician in Edinburgh. He was well known as the inventor of a locally used miner's safety lamp, and used his authority in Sunderland with great responsibility and coolness. He shared all the social prejudices, pressures and medical ignorance of his colleagues and yet refused to be panicked by the confusion at the end of October.

The Sunderland Board spent the summer seeking more information about cholera, recommending various sanitary measures and making sure that all the local medical profession would co-operate and be informed if the epidemic came. As part of their search for better information the Medical Board invited James Butler Kell, surgeon to the reserve division of the 82nd Regiment of Foot, to join the medical department of the Board. Kell had one major advantage over all other men in Sunderland. He had seen and treated cholera in Grant Port,

Mauritius in 1819-20 and 1829 whilst stationed there with the regiment.[1] In early June he addressed a meeting of the medical profession of Sunderland and impressed upon them the contagious nature of cholera. Kell had major disadvantages in Sunderland medical circles. He was a surgeon, which placed him in social status and authority well below all the physicians of the town. Further, he was an army surgeon, which placed him below those surgeons with local practices. He had no local connections – Sunderland had no experience of James Butler Kell, surgeon, that would enable them to judge how far his statements and recommendations could be accepted as reliable. He might claim to know more about cholera than anyone else, but how reliable was his insistence on quarantine, hospitals and separating the sick from the healthy? No one knew, and after the excitement of June and the tedium of waiting for ships held up in quarantine, no one paid much attention to him or to cholera. When Clanny called a meeting of the local medical profession in August to consider the reports from Russia, very few men attended.

During August several isolated cases occurred in Sunderland, any one of which might have been Asiatic cholera; a painter of earthenware named Allison, who lived two miles above the town (which was where the quarantine station was placed); an agricultural labourer who lived in the same area, John Lane, a quayside labourer, recovered in care of Mr Embleton, the parish surgeon. All had characteristic symptoms. The case which attracted Kell's attention was that of Robert Henry, a pilot, who guided a ship from the Baltic into the Wear in early August and piloted the ship out on the 12th. On the 14th he was dead, and his symptoms included severe cramps and blue nails on fingers and toes. His surgeon, a man named Cook, admitted several months later when he had had ample experience of cholera that this case was indeed Asiatic cholera.

Kell was sure at the time, but his attempts to rouse others to the fact indicate the disadvantages of a man without social status or authority. On 2 and 3 September he wrote to Sir James McGrigor on the Central Board of Health, obviously anticipating difficulties, for he wrote to the military man on the Board, trusting him more than Seymour, the physician who was Secretary. The London Board was not very excited and asked for more details. In a letter dated 8 September, Kell gave as much information as he knew. He tried to get more and passed the request from London to Clanny, who put the matter to the Sunderland Board which resolved 'to decline any interference on their part'.[2] The tension between Kell – probably regarded as an insignificant and meddling surgeon from the barracks – and the established medical

Sunderland 41

élite of Sunderland was building up. Kell had had his moment of importance in June and was not being allowed to stir up any more alarm. Meanwhile, Seymour had written to Sir Cuthbert Sharp, Collector of Customs at Sunderland to check other parts of Kell's story. On 8 September Kell gave Sharp all the details he could, and Sir Cuthbert sent a couple of tide-waiters to interview the surviving pilots of the Baltic ship on which Henry had travelled. They all denied having been on the ship — they had probably broken several quarantine regulations by leaving the ship so promptly. Kell heard no more of the matter until a casual meeting with Sir Cuthbert Sharp told him of the pilots' denial. Kell's campaign to have the presence of cholera in Sunderland acknowledged had been brought to a halt for over a month by the authorities starving him of information. Desperately he wrote to Sharp asking that the pilots be examined before a magistrate. This was refused.[3] There is now no means of knowing if Kell's suspicions about Robert Henry and his fellow pilot who had recovered were correct — Kell hadn't even seen the case. But it is certain that those in authority never gave Kell a fair chance to prove his point and never felt any sense of urgency about the reports he sent. Not that the Sunderland medical men felt they were ignoring the cholera. On 2 September the medical committee of the local Board had met and agreed to form district visiting committees which inspected their area and advised the authorities on much-needed cleansing measures.[4] All this gave an appearance of soothing and responsible preparation. To publish the existence of cholera in Sunderland had no part in the advice being given by the medical journals and official circulars.

In October and early November events moved with increasing speed. A community which felt it had done as well as any to prepare for cholera looked foolish and confused at the crucial moment.

9 October Robert Joyce of Cumberland Street, Bishopwearmouth, became ill with vomiting, purging cramps and cold skin. His surgeon Mr Dixon reported the matter to the medical committee, who thanked him and decided, 'there do not exist at present reasons for communicating them [the facts of the case] to the Board of Health.'[5] In retrospect, both Dixon and Clanny, who visited the case, were sure that this was Asiatic cholera.

17 October Isabella Hazard, twelve-year-old daughter of a respectable publican of Low Street, near the Fish Quay, was attacked. Despite the attention of Mr Cook, parish surgeon, she died within 24 hours. This case was important for two reasons. The house was only a short distance from the Sproats', and Clanny admitted that he found out about this case some three months later. The medical profession in Sunderland was so ill-co-ordinated and ill-informed about each other's doings that the local authority surgeon failed to pass vital information to the senior man in charge of anti-cholera measures. Despite the committees and meetings the profession largely acted as individuals in isolation. Still, even if Cook had recognised the case as Asiatic, he may have been deterred from reporting it by the cool reaction to Dixon's report earlier in the month.

23 October The case of William Sproat senior; Kell visited him with Dr Clanny, but only after declining an invitation from the keelman's wife because another surgeon, Mr Holmes, was already in attendance. Kell was careful to maintain professional etiquette when the risk of local hostility was so great. Kell stated that the Sproat case was Asiatic cholera and Clanny agreed.

27 October Both Sproat junior and his daughter were ill. Kell wrote to McGrigor again, and was instrumental in getting Robinson the chief magistrate to write to Melbourne, and, through Clanny, in moving the two Sproats into the Infirmary for their care and the public safety.

28 October A meeting of medical men at the Infirmary saw the two patients and stated that 'it was the common cholera of this country attended with aggravated symptoms,'[6] despite Kell stating his belief that it was Asiatic; this meeting took place before any social pressure had had time to develop.

29 October Kell wrote again to McGrigor with more details of Sproat's symptoms, and telling him of the disagreement with the rest of the Sunderland medical profession. Kell was not invited to visit the Infirmary – he could not go in by right because he was not elected to any of the consultant posts. Thus the man with the necessary experience was again cut off from the crucial sources of knowledge he needed.

31 October Two isolated cases, a shoemaker and a keelman.

1 November Eliza Turnbull, a nurse at the Infirmary who had helped remove the body of Sproat junior, suffered an appalling attack in the early hours of the morning and was dead by afternoon. This

Sunderland 43

well-publicised case caused great alarm in the town despite subsequent attempts to attribute her death to fear of cholera rather than cholera itself.[7]

A well-attended meeting of the Board of Health agreed that 'spasmodic cholera prevailed in Sunderland', and sent official notification to the government and the London Board of Health.

2 November The distrustful Kell, who must have been feeling increasingly helpless watching from the sidelines, again wrote to Sir James McGrigor. Ill temper, a product of the tension between Kell's inferior social and professional status and his superior knowledge of cholera, had already crept into his relationships with the rest of Sunderland, for his letter regretted an earlier 'hasty' letter, which had been a complaint against the imperfect quarantine administration at Sunderland. This time Kell contented himself with confirming that the cases of the keelman, his son and daughter were indeed Asiatic cholera. He also took care to inform the Sunderland Board of Health that he was writing so that no one could accuse him of going behind their backs. The friendly restraining hand of the senior army medical man must have prevented Kell's anger and frustration at the treatment he was receiving, earning him more ill will than it did in Sunderland.[8]

3 November Mrs Wilson, 22, daughter of a previous victim, was taken ill in one of the better parts of Sunderland.

4 November A correspondent of the *Courier* in London reported from Newcastle that Asiatic cholera was in Sunderland. For the first time the news from Sunderland was available for general public discussion outside the north-east of England.

5 November The first agent of the central government arrived in Sunderland. This was Dr Daun, a half-pay army surgeon with Indian experience of cholera. He was one of the men who had given evidence to the Central Board of Health earlier in the year. With Kell and Clanny, he visited Mrs Wilson and confirmed that hers was a case of Asiatic cholera. The government now had a source of information in Sunderland, which was not influenced by local fears and suspicions. Sunderland also had for the first time a member of its anti-cholera organisation who was concerned with national as well as local interests.

6 November Several new cases were recorded, a pilot, a sailor, a surgeon and Mrs Haslewood, a physician's wife. She had unwisely been present at the dissection of the nurse who had died in the Infirmary.

The same day, Lieutenant-Colonel Creagh, another half-pay army man, arrived from London armed with the limited amount of authority which the Privy Council, under the quarantine laws, could give him. A letter from Clanny told him that six new cases of cholera had been reported to the medical faculty meeting at three that afternoon. Creagh promptly ordered a 15-day quarantine on all vessels leaving the Wear, a course of action anticipated by his masters in London. The draft of the quarantine order in the Privy Council papers was dated 4 November, the day Creagh would have left for London.[9]

7 November (Monday) There were three more cases. Sunderland was visited by a medical deputation sent by the Mayor of Newcastle. The same day, on the advice of Kell, the gates of the barracks were closed, and the only contact which the men of the 82nd had with the rest of the community was through a few trusted individuals who collected supplies. The regiment had no cholera cases.

8 November There were at least three more cases. The Newcastle deputation reported to its own Board that the Sunderland disease was not imported and was not of foreign origin.[10]

9 November A meeting of magistrates, ship-owners and principal inhabitants was held at the Exchange, Sunderland. Clanny told them that the cholera was increasing, and they subscribed liberally to a fund for the relief of the poorer classes, but could not agree on setting up a cholera hospital because no one wanted the building in their area.[11]

10 November (Thursday) A meeting was held in the magistrates' room at the Exchange consisting of the principal inhabitants, some members of the medical profession, the High Sheriff of the County, and the Chief Magistrate in the chair. Despite hearing Dr Daun's views, the meeting cast doubt upon the presence of Asiatic cholera in Sunderland, and censured those medical men who had reported cases of the disease to London. Kell found the meeting especially unfriendly to him, and decided to withdraw from public affairs in Sunderland. The reason for the hostility was obvious. He was an outsider and the only name to be published in the London *Courier's* reports of cholera in Sunderland. The meeting wanted the names of the other doctors who had signed the report to the government, but never got this information.[12]

Sunderland 45

After the initial shock the commercial interests of Sunderland were becoming increasingly indignant about the restrictions on the coal trade. The commander of the naval sloop stationed at the mouth of the river was a man of irritating energy and firmness. He fired a shot ahead of any ship which left the Wear and attempted to ignore his orders, thus forcing the ship to turn back.[13] Annoyance was increased by the realisation that no cases were occurring on the ships in quarantine, and that the mail coaches ran freely to London in 36 hours, whilst the colliers were banned from the salt water passage. It was absurd and it was expensive.[14] Several surgeons were none too pleased on their own account, for they held shares in local shipping. Ships were traditionally owned in 1/64ths or 1/32nd shares. Thus professional men and tradesmen, often men of small means, could become part of the shipping interest.[15]

11 November (Friday) There were two tense meetings in Sunderland, closely followed by a third. The first took place in the afternoon at the Exchange. The meeting agreed that the much-publicised deaths of recent weeks had been 'common bowel complaints', and were not Indian cholera and were not of foreign origin. They attacked the reports in the *Courier,* dated Newcastle, as 'wicked and malicious falsehood', and condemned 'any individual' who had reported Indian cholera to the government, whatever his motives.

A further and more vicious meeting was held in the evening. This began by asking for a meeting of the medical profession at noon next day, to report the profession's opinion concerning the presence of cholera in the town. The meeting then resolved to obtain all correspondence between the Sunderland Board of Health and London and then publish the names of all medical practitioners who had reported cases of Asiatic cholera. The implied threat to men who relied on fee-paying patients or ratepayer-controlled poor law appointments for their income was clear.

Clanny, perhaps by design, had absented himself from the emotive pressures of the Friday meeting, but he was back for the calmer meeting in the sanctuary of the Infirmary on Saturday, and his influence was evident in a carefully worded statement put out by that meeting. This statement and the public statements of the medical men at the Friday meeting received wide publicity.[16] Many contemporaries and historians have seen these statements as an extraordinary and dishonest denial of the presence of Asiatic cholera in Sunderland, made in complete contradiction of the evidence and of the resolution of 1 November, and made under irresponsible though perhaps understandable pressure from selfish commercial interests. The *Edinburgh Medical and Surgical Journal* abandoned its usual measured tones and accused the Sunderland doctors of a deliberate attempt to deceive government and Press 'under the impulse of strong private interest'. The *Lancet* as usual was more outspoken.

> We will not speak of the conduct of many practitioners in Sunderland in those terms of reprobation which we think it so well deserves. That a posse of starving colliers should threaten to 'burn the doctors' who dare to admit the existence of the disease in that town is scarcely a matter of surprise; but that there should be found a set of well educated men weak enough to pander to the clamorous prejudices of the populace, is almost beyond credibility. Taking leave of them for the present, we solicit their attention to the 'Proclamation' which their conduct has elicited, and which points out the heavy responsibility incurred by medical men who venture to endanger the public safety by thwarting the precautions it requires when threatened by so appalling a calamity as the spreading of a pestilential epidemic.[17]

Pressures there certainly were. The threat of the colliers was no mean threat. The Sunderland mob had a reputation for selective and effective destruction when they felt their just interests were threatened. In 1815, the keelmen and casters had pulled down a new bridge, staithe and spout which Messrs Nesham had unwisely built to bring the coal wagons further into the port and hence rob the keelmen of some of their work. The following year another mob had attacked the grocers' shops which had refused to accept worn coin.[18]

The internal pressures of the commercial community of Sunderland were backed up by the work of the coal-owners of the surrounding countryside. These men were led by the large landowners who based their power and fortunes on the royalties and profits of the mines which had been developed on their estates. The coal-owners did not watch the imposition of quarantine regulations with the same calm as the cloth men. The coal trade needed the steady flow of colliers down the east coast to their major market in London. The textile manufacturers might survive the stop in trade through the stocks of raw material they held in their warehouses. The coal-owners faced falling profits on their massive capital investment, and the risk of discontented unemployed colliers, casters and keelmen. Sir Hedworth Williamson, Bart, head of an

established family which had lived at Whitburn Hall to the north of
Sunderland for several generations, and made its money from coal as
well as land, wrote directly to Viscount Melbourne, just as his status as
a major landowner and deputy lieutenant of the County entitled him to
do. He told Melbourne that the Sunderland disease was limited in
extent and did not appear to be infectious, though admittedly it had
the same symptoms as Asiatic cholera. He reported the discontent of
the ship-owners, merchants and traders of Sunderland with inconsistent
regulations that stopped trade by sea but not by land and warned,

> The lower orders will suffer most severely from want of employment
> and their poverty will be another cause of the increase of sickness
> and render them turbulent and riotous.[19]

One section of the ruling class was using the threat of riot against
another section of their class to protect the profit and wages of a
sectional economic interest. The Marquis of Londonderry, perhaps the
wealthiest of the Durham coal-owners, had just returned to his seat at
Wynyard Park, some 20 miles from Sunderland, after doing his part to
halt the progress of the Reform Bill. The Sunderland mob had burnt
his effigy, along with that of a bishop, after a town meeting to support
the Bill. If he differed from Sunderland on politics, their interest in
trade was identical. Londonderry depended on coal revenues to pay the
debts he had incurred by building Seaham Harbour, and to maintain the
princely style of life which he had created for himself.[20] He wrote to
the London *Standard* to calm the public mind about the reports from
Sunderland. He enclosed a letter from Dr J. Brown of Sunderland, an
old army medical officer who had served in the Peninsular War with
Londonderry, and who thus might owe him more than feudal loyalty.
Brown's views were much the same as those of Hedworth Williamson.[21]
Londonderry was not playing quite straight with Sunderland, for he
wrote privately to Sir William Pym saying that the ship *Surtees* on
which cholera had been reported had contracted the disease at
Sunderland, and that he had now cut contact between Sunderland and
Seaham, so could he have the quarantine on Seaham lifted?[22] In public,
Vane Londonderry still maintained his faith in Sunderland by
remaining with his family at Wynyard Park, exposed, he claimed, to the
same risks as the rest of the population. Still, he was used to taking
risks: his style of duelling was to receive his opponent's fire then
discharge his own weapon into the air.[23]

In the light of the pressures and criticisms directed at them, the statements of the Sunderland medical profession need careful examination. The commercial men were very clear in their denial of cholera at the afternoon meeting, but they had never claimed that the disease existed. The reports from India and Russia had led them to expect that cholera, once it arrived, would spread with sudden and disastrous speed, whilst the Sunderland disease spread in a slow and halting fashion. The doctors were vague and quarantine was damaging local trade. If Sunderland was attempting to conceal anything, then local actions were very odd. The *Sunderland Herald* published the fact that five unusual cases of common bowel complaints had occurred in the town and the Friday meetings gave further national publicity to those cases. When the *Times* reporter arrived in Sunderland on the 13th he found everything normal. The theatre was open. A recent meeting about a proposed wet dock had been well attended. Local people were not behaving as if a dangerous epidemic was amongst them. They were not concealing cholera. They just did not believe that it existed. As the reporter neared Sunderland, he found people more and more prepared to discount the cholera. The confusion was in part a result of the manner in which most of the population had been prepared for the arrival of cholera. The information in the Press had been at worst sensational and at best anticipating large-scale epidemic, with hints that it might all never happen. Nothing prepared people for the initial first-cases phase of the epidemic. Sunderland found the precautions expensive, the threat hard to discern, and decided that the small risk did not justify the heavy cost.

The behaviour of the medical profession at the Friday evening and the Saturday meeting on first examination appeared to warrant the accusations of dishonesty and weakness in the face of social pressure, especially as these meetings reversed the decision of the 1 November meeting. The published statements of the men at the evening meeting were not as simple as this. A few men did deny the existence of cholera in Sunderland. Most were more careful and said the cases were 'aggravated English cholera'. It was understandable that surgeon Dixon should feel this way. When he had reported a case in early October as Asiatic cholera he was politely ignored by the medical faculty of the local Board of Health. According to the *Tyne Mercury* two men did acknowledge the presence of cholera in Sunderland. Mr Torbuck stated, 'a cholera has appeared in the town of a malignant character, such as has never been known in this town before, either as it regards the symptoms before death, during the progress of the disease, or on examination after death; but not of a contagious or infectious character.'

Torbuck should have known, for Haslewood and Mordey recorded that he was case number ten in the Sunderland epidemic on 6 November — a remarkable recovery in order to attend the meeting on the 11th; had he really had Asiatic cholera? Mr Penman, who was believed to have been the house surgeon on duty at the Infirmary when Sproat was brought in, told the meeting, 'The cholera which is now in town has the same symptoms as that which has appeared in foreign countries and is infectious.'[24] Others admitted a serious disease, but all were of one opinion, with the exception of Penman, that whatever it was, it was not contagious.

The statement issued by the Saturday meeting needs full quotation and commentary, for it showed exactly what the medical men of Sunderland were doing.

> Resolved — that a disease possessing every symptom of epidemic cholera is now existing in this town; [that was true and contradicted nothing said at the 1 November meeting and nothing said by Kell] that it has never appeared on board of ships; [again true, or at least no record existed of cases on board ship] that there is not the slightest ground for imagining that it has been imported, [debatable, Kell certainly would have contested this point if he had been unwise enough to appear and speak at the meeting] nor has it extended itself by contagion, though the sufferers have been attended by numbers of friends and neighbours [debatable again, one nurse and a surgeon were already in the record books as victims — still their cases were being explained in other ways].
> That it appears to have arisen from atmospherical distemperature [accords well with much contemporary medical thought including that of Reid Clanny who signed the resolution] acting in most cases on persons weakened by want of wholesome food and clothing, by bad air, intemperance or previous disease; [this fully agreed with the line taken in official reports] and that the interruption of the commerce of the port seems to offer the most probable means of extending the disease, by depriving the industrious poor of their bread, and thus placing their families in the depths of misery and distress. [Here then was the centre of the problem, but still a very reasonable statement from those who believed that poverty increased the propensity to develop these 'symptoms'.]
> In conclusion, the medical gentlemen trust that the above statements will remove any misconstructions and false reports which have arisen out of this unpleasant affair; and beg to congratulate

their fellow townsmen on the otherwise good health of the town.

The *Tyne Mercury* for one understood what was intended,

> It is true this [the denial of cholera] is not stated in express terms. The language is vague, general and guarded, and though it might admit of a different construction, the obvious one intended is the non-existence at Sunderland of Asiatic Cholera.

But as many observers asked, what did the doctors of Sunderland think they were doing, admitting that a disease with the same symptoms as Asiatic cholera was in the town, but claiming that the disease was not Asiatic cholera? Their action made sense only in terms of the inconclusive controversy between contagionists and non-contagionists. Several Sunderland doctors, including Clanny and Brown, had been non-contagionists, even before the cholera. Sunderland knew that contagion meant quarantine, and that quarantine meant commercial dislocation, unemployment and increased poverty, with little obvious gain to the town or the rest of the country. In October 1831, it was impossible to assert that cholera was not contagious. Contagion and cholera were firmly associated in the public and political mind which the Sunderland meeting was trying to influence, so the doctors of Sunderland tried to outflank the political victory of the contagionists and decided that their symptoms should not be called Asiatic cholera. Identifying the same set of symptoms as two different diseases, one contagious and the other not, was not a new idea, for McGrigor had done this in his work on yellow fever. The Sunderland doctors' statement of 12 November was a neat balancing act which did full justice to the facts as then understood and took account of local community pressures. This was done not by dishonesty but by taking advantage of the inconclusive state of the scientific debate on contagion.

Whilst these meetings were taking place Dr Daun was getting the local cholera administration into shape. He was joined shortly after his arrival by Dr Gibson, a young doctor from Edinburgh whom he praised as 'a willing and able assistant'. Gibson worked hard despite the continual worry that the government would not pay him enough to compensate for the loss of private practice in Edinburgh. Later in the month the government men were joined by Dr Barry who brought direct European experience to the north-east. Daun and Gibson did three jobs as government representatives in Sunderland. They helped with local administrative organisation. Daun encouraged the Sunderland Board of

Sunderland 51

Health to divide the town into districts for the provision of medicines and medical attendance. He also pressed the authorities to set up a cholera hospital to isolate cases from the rest of the population. In his initial haste Daun made the insensitive and tactless proposal that the Assembly rooms, a major middle-class meeting place, should be used. But through the efforts of the Rev. Mr Grey, the Rector of Sunderland, a small schoolroom was obtained.[25] The second task was to provide a flow of regular and reliable information for London. This was not easy. They had to overcome the natural aversion which all doctors had against revealing details of their patients' illness. Daun rebuked the local doctors for concealing cases from him. They had 'a desire to call the disease of their patients by any other name than cholera'. To counter this Daun divided his returns into diarrhoea, common (English) cholera and Asiatic cholera, which only served to reduce their social and political impact in the early days.[26] Some omissions arose from simple confusion for Clanny told Seymour (secretary to the Central Board and another physician) that he thought Daun was dealing with all reports.[27] Finally, the government men attended patients and helped the overtaxed local doctors.

Daun and Gibson were free of local pressures but they were still hampered by the social structure of their own profession. They had grown up in a profession which was becoming increasingly jealous of its status as a body of qualified men. As soon as the cholera hospital was established, the Sunderland Board of Health appointed the parish surgeon to look after it. This was the cheapest thing they could do as he was already employed by the parish, but he was an apothecary who practised as a surgeon, 'that sort of half-educated practitioner with whom Dr. Gibson and I would find it very unpleasant to act', as Daun told Pym. Despite this initial hostility Embleton settled down at the cholera hospital and gained especial note for his courtesy and help to the many doctors who came to Sunderland to learn about cholera.[28] Daun himself became particularly exasperated with the inability of the local medical men to co-operate. He was a military man used to accounting for what he was doing within a bureaucratic structure. 'You have no idea', he told Pym on the 11th, 'how difficult it is to drill the civil medicos in anything like method in sending me their reports and I fear that a few of them are doing it not very willingly'. Daun found the magistrates wishing to do what was right but lacking in power. He also had to work in the shadow of a large local Board of Health of merchants and ship-owners, a 'motley assembly...where all is noise and dispute', and he resolved 'to have nothing to do with it'.

The most intractable problem of all in Sunderland was poverty. The government was alarmed and its agents were shocked by what they found. Soon after his arrival Barry wrote a detailed report to Pym. Significantly, he emphasised that it was not an official letter, 'lest it might come out with my name, before I can escape from here. The black diamond merchants would condemn me to the mines for such a suggestion...'. Suspicion between local people and the government agents was growing.

Sunderland as an economic and social unit consisted of three parishes, Sunderland itself, down by the river, Bishopwearmouth on the higher ground south of the river and Monkwearmouth across the bridge to the north. Barry described the dynamic of their social geography with some precision.

> Sunderland contains almost exclusively the working poor, with their parents, wives and children, many of whom disease and age renders incapable of earning their own subsistence. They live in crowded dwellings and are most strikingly disproportionate in numbers to those capable of paying parish rates. The assessable persons in the parish are chiefly composed of shopkeepers, low traders, incipient speculators, and others of small uncertain incomes... As soon as a man, who has himself perhaps commenced as a labourer, feels that he can live at ease, he retires to the parish of Bishopwearmouth, which comprises the elevated part of the town, wide clean streets, the grand houses; – in short the west end.

Thus the parish system of caring for the poor, originally devised to ensure that a community took responsibility for its own poor, was being used by the wealthier inhabitants of Sunderland to avoid their responsibilities. Barry wanted the two parishes of Sunderland and Bishopwearmouth united,

> The rich would thus be obliged to preserve from starvation and premature decay, the very instruments by which their fortunes were built, but which in this place they desert when their fortunes reach a certain bulk.

Barry held a traditional view of social responsibility. He wanted the ruling class or government to step into a local situation to force the middle classes of society to do their duty towards the poor. There was no prospect of using legal pressure in November. The government contented itself with subscribing £50 to a fund for the relief of the sick and distressed which by the end of the month was said to amount to £1,300.[29]

Despite the threat to use troops in the 20 October regulations, there was no effective move to impose internal quarantine on Sunderland. The Central Board considered and rejected the idea.[30] The mayors of Stockton and Staindrop and the authorities of Barnard Castle forbade the carriers' carts from Sunderland to enter their towns. Stockton constituted its Board of Health for this very purpose.[31] The Bishop of Durham asked Sunderland to limit contact with the rest of the county and was promptly visited by a deputation from the town, who told him that the danger was small. The Bishop decided that agitation in the county was great enough to call a county meeting which took place on the 21st and decided, with the aid of some hard talking from the Marquis of Londonderry, that no restrictions were necessary.[32]

Meanwhile, Poulett-Thompson had told the House of Commons that surrounding Sunderland with a *cordon sanitaire* 'could have been done only with the most injurious and vexatious consequences to the town and neighbourhood, and would have proved utterly ineffectual'. Even those with strong contagionist views admitted that English traditions of freedom would not allow the strong measures which had been tried (and had failed) in the more autocratic society of Russia.[33]

There were several weaknesses in the social structure and organisation of Sunderland which enabled cholera to enter Britain with such leisurely ease. The main weakness was the basic need of a commercial community to maintain the free flow of trade. All attempts to control the movement of ships and people out of and into Sunderland were opposed by political means, by scientific dispute, by main force and deception. Sunderland hampered all attempts to impose administrative controls upon itself in the early days of the epidemic. All sections of society took part. The keelmen used threats of violence. The merchants and professional men used their meetings, petitions, prevarication and argument. The aristocrats, Londonderry and Hedworth-Williamson, used their position within the ruling class. Sunderland's unwillingness to act against cholera was not due to class tensions or divisions. It was due to the solidarity of interests involved in the coal trade. The major weakness created by class conflict in Sunderland was the lack of provision for the poor. The conflict between the ratepayer and the poor had in part been resolved by the wealthier ratepayers' escape to the neighbouring parishes. The conflict between the ratepayers and the government, which wanted to see the middle class take responsibility for their poor, could not be resolved because of the government's lack of power in the localities.

Another major weakness was the imperfect development of medicine as a profession. Their independence of judgement was weakened by their reliance on the fees of patients who were also ratepayers and deeply involved in the shipping interest. Their power of action was further weakened by their lack of effective organisation amongst themselves. Those with honorary posts at the Infirmary and their social equals met in the Board of Health but had little liaison with the parish surgeons and apothecaries who served the poorer sections of society where cholera first appeared. Most crucial was the doctors' imperfect understanding of cholera which added genuine confusion to social pressure. This was not only a matter of contagion or otherwise, but also a matter of the identity of cholera itself. The doctors had long been used to dealing with a series of savage bowel complaints which they called English cholera. The medical literature contained accounts of an epidemic in Clapham in 1829 and Leeds in 1825, with symptoms of vomiting, purging and convulsion, and the massive loss of fluid and consequent cramps which were associated with cholera.[34] Many doctors believed that what they saw in Sunderland was only a severe form of the 'native' disease. It only needed a little social pressure and the fear of quarantine to convince them.

The central government was itself weak in the localities. The enquiries, plans and regulations were of little value without an adequate, efficient and powerful executive agency in the areas affected by cholera. The weakness showed first among the customs officials who were supposed to administer the June quarantine regulations. They were accused of 'culpable negligence' by the London papers, but their task was really an impossible one. Sunderland did not even have a suitable place to hold ships in quarantine. They could not be kept for long outside the river mouth because of the liability of strong on-shore winds which would have driven them ashore, so when a ship from a quarantine port arrived it was led up the river by its pilot to an anchorage called Deptford. a mile or so above the bridge. This was a place many of the colliers used when laid up during the winter. Here the ships remained with very little guard. It was reported that the crews of three ships from Hamburg, which many believed were the origin of the October cases, were able to ramble ashore each night of their stay.[35] No one ever established exactly how cholera did get ashore. It may have come from the Hamburg ships or the Riga flax boats in August. Some said it came from chests of clothes belonging to persons who had died of cholera in the Baltic, and these had arrived in the town in August.[36] Whatever the

Sunderland

reason, the quarantine measures were ineffective.

The apathetic reactions of the local board were understandable in terms of confusion and local interest. The slow reactions of the Central Board need a different explanation. Kell's first letter was read by the Board of Health in London on 5 September, yet Dr Daun did not arrive in Sunderland until 5 November, two months and several letters later. When the London Board received Kell's two letters to McGrigor about the August deaths, 'with symptoms supposed by the writer to resemble the cholera of Russia', they acted with a lack of urgency which was not surprising in light of a summer spent chasing false alarms. There was little in Kell's reports to distinguish it from the others. In July, Dr John Marshall had reported with great urgency from Glasgow that a violent cholera-like epidemic had broken out in the area around one of the local flax mills. He was sure that cholera had been imported with the Riga flax just as everyone had feared. One of the first to die lived 'precariously' for the sake of supporting his parents in Ireland, and 'he was in the habit of spending much of his idle time amongst the girls employed in the flax mill, and that Nancy Kitchen and he in particular had for some time lived in the closest intimacy.' She was also among the dead. Dr Daun was sent to Glasgow but by the end of the month had written to say it was only common cholera.[37] On 14 August they were told that a soldier in the barracks at Hull had died after 17 hours of cholera-like sickness, which included spasmodic movements of the abdominal muscles which the surgeon of the 7th Fusiliers took as the key symptom. Mahoney, the surgeon, locked all the troops in the barracks because of the alarm in the town. He found that this only increased the alarm so let them all out again, by which time Daun had arrived to say he had no reason to eliminate Asiatic cholera, but as there were no new cases there was nothing to worry about. After a summer checking false alarms from Leith to Margate, the Central Board was quite unable to identify the real one when it came. The Board had devised an administrative structure to deal with cholera when it arrived but failed to devise a rapid and effective method of identifying the first cases when they came ashore.

By the end of November, Sunderland had lost the battle to prove that cholera was not in the town. The epidemic lasted into January by which time 179 people were dead out of 368 cases. A milder visitation in the early summer brought the totals to 215 out of 554 cases.[38] This figure produced a relatively high death rate of 1.26 per cent, when compared with the population of Sunderland town as the Privy Council did, but a better comparison with the parliamentary borough of

Sunderland, which was the area from which the cases were drawn, produced a death rate of 0.25 per cent, well down the death tables of the cholera towns.

Notes

1. Kell, *Cholera at Sunderland*, appendix XII, p.105.
2. Ibid., p.27.
3. Ibid., p.28.
4. Clanny, *Cholera in Sunderland*, p.14.
5. Ibid., p.16.
6. Kell, *Cholera at Sunderland*, pp.34-5.
7. Ibid., p.36.
8. James Butler Kell to Sir James McGrigor, 2 November 1831, P.R.O., P.C.1/103.
9. Quarantine order on Sunderland vessels, P.R.O., P.C.1/103.
10. *Courier*, 14 and 15 November 1831, quoting the *Tyne Mercury* as well as their own correspondent in Newcastle.
11. Kell, *Cholera at Sunderland*, p.40.
12. Ibid., p.41.
13. *Courier*, 14 November 1831.
14. *Times*, 14 November 1831.
15. *Courier*, 13 November 1831.
16. *Sunderland Herald*, 12 November 1831; *Courier*, 14 November 1831; *Times*, 15 November 1831.
17. *E.M.S.J.*, vol.37, 1832, p.195; *Lancet*, 26 November 1831, p.309.
18. William Fordyce, *The History and Antiquities of the County Palatine of Durham. . .*, 2 vols., Newcastle 1857, vol.2, p.403.
19. Hedworth-Williamson to Melbourne, Whitburn Hall, 14 November 1831, P.R.O., P.C.1/103.
20. *Courier*, 26 October 1831; Sir Archibald Alison, *Lives of Lord Castlereagh and Sir Charles Stewart*, 3 vols., London, 1859, vol.3, pp.244-5.
21. *Times*, 16 November 1831.
22. Vane Londonderry to Sir William Pym, Wynyard Park, 27 November 1831, P.R.O., P.C. 1/103.
23. Edith H.V.T. Stewart, *Francis Anne*, London, 1958, pp.173-4.
24. *Courier*, 15 November 1831; Kell, *Cholera at Sunderland*, p.48.
25. Daun to Pym, Sunderland, 11 and 14 November 1831, P.R.O., P.C.1/103.
26. Daun to Pym, Sunderland, 15 November 1831. loc. cit.; *Times*, 22 November 1831.
27. Clanny to Seymour, Sunderland 15 November 1831, loc. cit.
28. Daun to Pym, Sunderland 15 November 1831, loc. cit.; *Lancet*, 26 November 1831.
29. Barry to Pym, Sunderland, 28 November 1831, P.R.O., P.C.1/103; Minutes of the Central Board of Health (fair copies), 26 November 1831, P.R.O., P.C.1/105.
30. Central Board of Health Letter Book to James Jobling Esq., Morpeth, 17 November 1831, P.R.O., P.C.1/93.
31. Loc. cit., 9 December 1831.
32. Kell, pp.66-7; *Times*, 21 and 24 November 1831.
33. *Hansard's Parliamentary Debates*, 3rd Series, vol.9, 1831-2, 15 December 1831; *Times*, 11 November 1831.
34. *London Medical and Physical Journal*, vol.62, 1829, p.281; Charles Turner Thackrah, *Cholera, its character and treatment. . .with reference to the disease*

as now existing in Newcastle and neighbourhood, London, 1832; *E.M.S.J.*, vol.29, 1828, p.71.
35. *Courier*, 5 November 1831.
36. *Lancet*, 4 February 1832, p.670.
37. Central Board of Health Minute Book, July 1831, P.R.O., P.C.1/101.
38. *London Medical Gazette*, 31 March 1831.

4 CONTAINMENT FAILS

The events in Sunderland showed that the Central Board of Health in London hoped to contain any spread of cholera in Britain by the active co-operation of rate-raising and rate-spending Local Boards of Health, guided by medical officers employed by the Central Board. Between October 1831 and May 1832 the Central Board employed some twenty medical men to provide a link between the centre and the localities. There were several army men like Daun and Creagh. These included four Deputy Inspectors General of Hospitals — Daun, James Arthur, John Maling and J.A. Knipe. The Board thus gained experienced senior men for 3s. a day travelling allowance and 21s. per week lodging allowance. They were intensively used until June. In the last six weeks (for which the accounts survive) they cost £113. A number of less senior men were employed for shorter periods, a staff surgeon, a regimental surgeon and a man from Ordnance. These men were relatively more expensive. They were on half pay and entitled to higher rates of subsistence, and cost £167.2s.11d. in the same six-week period. The June accounts include six civilians, men like Simeon Bullen, Thurston Caton and William Rennie, who were active in Scotland, and cost £31.1s.0d. each over the six-week period, which included 10s.6d. for lodging and 7s.6d. per day. This, with the expenses of two full-pay naval surgeons, brought the Central Board's salary bill up to £474.9s.10d. for the period 1 April-15 May 1832. The totals in the previous two months, before the Board's campaign in the field began to run down, had been £526.11s.10d. and £428.7s.10d.[1]

In Sunderland and Newcastle and especially in Scotland, these men were used to supervise the work of the local boards, to advise, cajole and frighten these boards into providing adequate hospitals and medication, into finding and reporting cases, administering cleansing, and attempting to isolate suspects and quarantine local transport. The Central Board men, especially the junior and the civilian medical men, were sent to augment the local medical profession in places where it was weak or overtaxed. The senior men, in addition, provided London with one of the few independent sources of information which the government had on the progress of the disease. As they followed the cholera track in an attempt to make the government's anti-cholera policy effective in the localities, these men found themselves hampered by their lack of legal authority and by the needs and prejudices of the society they found.

I

After Sunderland, attention turned to Newcastle on the north bank of the Tyne. Newcastle made its money from exporting coal as well as from the ironworks, glassworks, potteries and shipbuilding yards along the river. The crowded houses of the sailors, keelmen, coal-casters and labourers who worked along the waterfront, especially in the narrow lanes or 'chares' which linked the upper part of the town with the Sandgate, were the perfect filthy ill-drained target for cholera. The mayor, Archibald Reed, with his eye on the possibility of quarantine on the trade of the Tyne, was clearly on the defensive. He wrote to the Privy Council in the early part of November assuring them of the health of the town and describing the cleansing measures taken.[2] Events in Newcastle followed a very similar pattern to those of Sunderland. There were a few scattered cases, some false alarms, others genuine and their implication ignored, and others which must never have been reported at all. In late October a man called Oswald Reay died with symptoms later recognised as 'denoting the disease in its worst form'. The body was examined by three leading medical men of the town who reported that it might be cholera but 'there has been no reason for believing that the cause of his death had a Foreign Origin.'[3] Death from an English disease was apparently less alarming. During November the Newcastle Board of Health intensified its activities, sending observers to Sunderland and cleansing the streets. The death of William Armstrong in early November caused another round of alarmed speculation. The body was examined by Messrs Headlam, Frost and Greenhow, who wrote to the mayor congratulating him on the opportunity they had for dispelling 'unfounded alarm'. This letter, like the report on the previous case, was immediately printed as a handbill and circulated. Other less serious souls placarded the walls with a poster appealing for cases to be reported,

> Any person supplying the Board of Health with a few cases of Asiatic Cholera, will receive a liberal and substantial reward; and should none such be obtainable, any number of cases of British origin, however small, will be thankfully received and most gratefully acknowledged...(the writers) trust...fellow townsmen...will endeavour by every means in their power, to get up a few Appearances, to save the Credit of the Firm from the sneers of the credulous, and

the aspertions of the ignorant and malicious.[4]

On 26 November, a labouring man called Robert Jordan was taken ill in the lower part of the town with 'stomach cramps'. The mayor, acting with a rare sense of duty, reported this case to the Privy Council as cholera. The Privy Council responded more rapidly than a month before and declared that ships leaving the Tyne should no longer have a clean bill of health and sent their medical officers north to investigate. Daun reported somewhat oddly that the symptoms of Jordan's case were such that had it been in Sunderland he would have called it malignant cholera. In the pause between Jordan's case and the next confirmed case the commercial interests of Newcastle met and censured the mayor for reporting to the Privy Council, but cholera had no respect for the politics of trade. On 7 December cholera was officially confirmed in Newcastle. The number of cases rose to a peak over the next few weeks and then faded, but Newcastle was not so fortunate as Sunderland. Cholera returned in the summer to leave the town in October 1832 with 801 deaths and 3,487 cases attributed to cholera, one of the worst records for a town of that size in the kingdom.[5]

Once established in the two major population centres of north-east England cholera spread slowly but persistently among the towns and villages of Northumberland and Durham. In the first week of December it reached the colliery districts of Hetton and Houghton-le-Spring. The same week, Denis McGuire, a mendicant dealer in old rags, walked from Sunderland to North Shields bringing cholera. The week before a man from the hamlet of Lemington on the north banks of the Tyne, west of Newcastle, had visited his son who was dying of cholera in Newcastle. He returned with the disease. There must have been countless such contacts, people visiting relatives, tramping for work and trading in the markets, any one of which could have spread cholera. By mid-December cholera had been reported in the collieries of Seghill, Wide Open and Backworth, as well as the low-lying and dirty ironworks village of Swalwell.[6] The colliery villages were especially vulnerable. The majority of the houses were two or three roomed, terraced and built in rows. They were cluttered with sheds for pigs and poultry. Though spacious by urban standards, their drainage and water supply was inadequate. Once the stream or the wells at the top of the village had become infected, the whole population was threatened. The working conditions of the miner were ideal for the spread of cholera for, as a later investigator was told, 'the pit is one vast privy' and the men, who ate but could not wash underground, passed the infection readily from one to another.

The epidemic was a disaster which crept up on the communities it affected. It moved slowly in the chill of winter. Most places began with a few scattered cases. Sometimes this was all. In others a reservoir of infection built up and a rapid spread of the disease followed.

The most alarming explosive epidemics of the winter were in Gateshead and Newburn. Newcastle excluded all vagrants from the city as part of their public health campaign. Most of these had simply taken refuge in Gateshead on the south bank of the river. Up to 25 December there had, surprisingly, been only two cases of cholera in Gateshead. But sometime on Christmas Day the water supply of the town must have become heavily infected. That evening and in the next two days cases occurred in terrifying numbers so that by ten o'clock on 27 December there had been 99 cases and 42 deaths. By the end of January 391 persons had been attacked and 141 killed. The final total was 148 dead and 407 cases in a population of 15,000.[7] Newburn stood on the north bank of the Tyne. Though the population of the parish was nearly 2,000. that of the village was only 550, mainly colliers, glassworkers and wherrymen. Although there was no apparent contact with infected villages, the first case occurred on 4 January in a low-lying house by the Newburn stream. Other scattered cases occurred in the same locality until 15 January when 14 new cases were reported including Mr Edmondson, the vicar, who had been noted for his care in avoiding infection. The next day there were 50 new cases. By 2 February, there had been 320 attacks and 55 deaths in the village population of 550. John Snow, in his mid-century investigation, blamed the Newburn disaster on the ironworks half a mile from the village which used the small stream as a privy. This seems a long distance for the infection to travel, but whatever means of entry cholera found to Newburn and Gateshead, once established in the water supply, it travelled with devastating speed. Both places were built on the sloping banks of the Tyne, where infection found it simple to travel from privy midden to well-head.[8]

Once alerted to the danger in the north-east of England the Central Board of Health put their medical agents into the field with all dispatch. Gibson moved to Houghton-le-Spring and then joined Daun and Creagh on the Tyne. Francis MacCann arrived in the colliery districts around Sunderland with two of the young civilians, Simeon Bullen and Thurston Caton. Their experience in the first few weeks was a warning of difficulties to come. In Newcastle, the hospital plans neatly set out in the circulars failed. Although 20 to 40 cases were reported each day, only three or four were brought to Sandgate hospital at the centre of the epidemic,

> the prejudice against which is so strong that nothing but the most abject poverty and destitution can overcome it and then rarely before the disease has existed some hours and the patient is in a state of collapse.[9]

In the large towns there was concealment, delay and a moderate amount of good will. The government men were appalled by the poverty of the population they sought to help, but could always turn to the resources of the wealthier members of the community for help as they did at Sunderland. In the smaller villages and the little ports along the Tyne, the medical men found poverty was caused not by the distribution of resources but by the total lack of them. Creagh, with some government money at his disposal, gave sundry amounts like the £50 at North Shields to encourage local contributions. Elsewhere on the Tyne, he was hampered in his task of setting up hospitals by the lack of bedding and applied to the barracks at Tynemouth for help. From Tynemouth he wrote in despair that the place was without even an apothecary's shop and even the troops there were without medical help.[10] Some of the stress of the situation was indicated in a letter which Gibson, Daun's able young assistant, wrote from Durham where he had been sent to investigate an isolated case. The man had died in Durham workhouse after coming from a lodging-house in Newcastle and being picked up drunk from the road. Dr Cooke saw him and decided cholera. Another doctor claimed drink was the cause of death. Gibson found Cooke was 'a great alarmist and appeared to me a little mad'. Cooke, it transpired, had written a great tract on cholera after visiting Sunderland for an hour, and Gibson suspected that the alarm was designed to boost sales. Back in Newcastle, Gibson raged against concealment, especially the activities of Mr Tim, surgeon, and the *Tyne Mercury*. The secretary of the Central Board returned the letters to Gibson as not fit to be entered in the minutes and warned him against future outbursts. Gibson apologised for the contents and in a few weeks returned to Edinburgh, worried about his family and private practice. Gibson was hard-working, something of an idealist and a realist, but not enough of a cynic to accept the realism of his fee-receiving, pamphlet-selling elders with the military calm of Daun, MacCann and Arthur.[11] If setting the medical defences of the Tyne and Wear was difficult and frustrating, the problems faced by Daun and Creagh were mild compared with those which met their colleague, James Arthur, further north. Experience in Scotland

II

In late December 1831, Major MacDonald found himself in Edinburgh to attend the court martial of a young dragoon who was accused of forging a letter. Major MacDonald was also one of the half-pay officers who had been appointed to the second Board of Health in November. His brief visit gave the Central Board an ideal opportunity for assuring Edinburgh of government support and of finding out a little of what was happening in Scotland. During his stay he visited Haddington, where cholera made its first appearance in Scotland on 17 December. No one established for sure how it got there. Some suggested that three cobblers who had walked from Newcastle were responsible. Haddington was on the Great North Road, a highway for coaches, carts, vagrants, pedlars and men tramping for work. There was ample opportunity for bringing the infection north. When the cholera was confirmed on the 25th, nearby Edinburgh received the news with alarm and consoled itself with the circumstances,

> The first case of cholera, which occurred on the 17th was a man extremely dissipated in his habits, who had been wandering about in a state of complete intoxication and almost naked the previous night.[12]

After a few days reflection the *Edinburgh Courant* realised that cholera was no worse than typhus. MacDonald visited Haddington with Drs Hamilton Bell and Meikle, both men with Indian experience and now members of the Edinburgh Board of Health. The three cobblers, he found, had arrived the day after the first case. Most of the cases were confined to the Nungate, 'a low and filthy part of the town', and he believed mostly among the dissipated. He attended the meetings of the Edinburgh Board of Health who regarded this as a special mark of respect. More reassuring to London must have been his reports on the preparations Edinburgh was making. There were handbills for informing the public, stations for the supply of medicine for early treatment, forms for recording all aspects of the disease and a committee for conducting a scientific investigation of the epidemic. MacDonald especially liked the arrangement for ten small hospitals instead of one large one for the whole city. The Edinburgh Board had even issued a memorandum which was delivered to all congregations in the city one

Containment Fails

Sunday in late November. It discussed the problem of the poor, especially liable to cholera because of their 'privations', with a degree of practicality that allowed no relaxation of moral censure,

> although a part of these privations and distresses among the poor may have been the result of their own improvidence, or habits of dissipation, yet a great part is the effect of unavoidable misfortune; and, at all events, while the lower orders continue so liable, as they unfortunately are, to the ravages of this epidemic disease, there can be no security against it extending itself widely among other classes of society.[13]

Major MacDonald returned to 'town' as soon as the court martial was over.

Haddington was an important market town, and once cholera was established there, isolated cases began to appear in the rural settlements of East Lothian, but cholera never gained a hold in places like Beanstone Mill, Athelstaneford and Whittinghame. The next major outbreak in Scotland was in the mining village of Tranent, a few miles further along the Edinburgh road. The most likely contact with Haddington was a beggar who died in a common lodging-house in the early days of the epidemic. The first cases on the 11th were followed by an explosive outbreak on the 18th. The eleven new cases included two colliers, a collier's wife, a coal-bearer, a woman who was taken ill in the pit, two labourers, a pauper, a hawker of crockery and a match-seller.[14] Cholera spread through the colliery and fishing villages that stretched along the south shore of the Firth of Forth. It was hastened on its way by the traditional holiday of Old Handsel Monday which came a fortnight after New Year, and was a time for visiting relatives, eating and drinking.[15] Cholera took its most explosive and violent form in the fishing village of Musselburgh. There were 447 cases and 202 deaths in a population of 7,800, mostly concentrated among the 1,500 people of Fisherrow. This was a close-knit fishing community related by many generations of intermarriage and by frequent day-to-day contact in the small, often windowless, houses that were crowded on the low-lying ground by the Forth. Visiting relatives brought cholera to Prestonpans (20 January) and Cockenzie (24 January).[16] By this time cholera was in the Borders, brought to Hawick by a cattle dealer who had visited the fair at Morpeth, where the disease had already been brought from Newcastle.[17]

The first Edinburgh cases were reported on 27 January. Both Edinburgh and Leith seem to have been infected and re-infected several times before the epidemic took hold in the crowded tenements of the capital. Most of the early cases were people who had visited relatives in the infected villages of East Lothian. The first to die in Leith was a cobbler, James Baxter. He had been with his sister to the funeral of another sister in Musselburgh. The Leith sister kissed the corpse as it lay in the coffin and she died before reaching home. Baxter himself died on 28 January.[18] Talk of non-contagion and the association of drink and cholera all served to make people less worried about infection and more concerned about their relatives, thus increasing contacts between the capital and surrounding villages.

The continual ebb and flow of vagrants and petty traders around the city added to the stream of infection. Among the first victims in Edinburgh was an Irish woman living in the West Bow who had been singing in the streets of Haddington, Musselburgh and Tranent, and then the Widow MacMillan, whose son, a hawker, had just returned from Musselburgh.[19]

On 2 February 1832, James Arthur, Deputy Inspector General of Hospitals, received his instructions from William MacLean, secretary to the Board of Health in Whitehall. He was to proceed to Glasgow and Kirkintilloch, 'You will assist by every means in your power to arrest the spread and diminish the mortality of cholera. . .' He was also to observe the pathology and clinical history of the disease. It was a formidable task for his responsibilities covered the counties of Lanark, Ayr, Stirling and Dunbarton. James Arthur's instructions were a consequence of the appearance of cholera in the west of Scotland. The first case occurred on 22 January at Kirkintilloch on the Grand Junction Canal which ran from the Forth to the Clyde. A boy called McMillan was taken ill in church and died the next day. It was easy to point to the canal as a possible source of contact with the east — some claimed that a boat from Newcastle with a load of hooves and hides was the boy's contact — but no one ever established the source of infection. This case was followed by others in the same area of the village. The Glasgow Board of Health promptly stationed their agents on the road to stop travellers coming from Kirkintilloch and Coatbridge, the next village to be infected. There was little they could do. Two coaches went to and from Kirkintilloch each day and as many of the population were weavers dependent on the manufacturers of Glasgow for their work and wages, they made frequent trips to the city. The canal operators were a little more co-operative and arranged for boats to be towed through the infected area by steam rather than horse so that the men on the boats would have no contact with shore. Such efforts were tokens of concern which had little effect on the flow of social and economic contact which brought cholera to Glasgow. The first acknowledged case was that of Janet Lindsay, an old asthmatic woman, very much addicted to drink, who lived in Todd's Close in the Goosedubbs, one of the most crowded and filthy areas of Glasgow. This was on 9 February. In the next few days scattered cases were reported in many parts of the city and the villages along the Clyde. The Glasgow epidemic was the worst in the kingdom. There were between 3,005 and 3,166 deaths according to different sources, over 1,000 of them in the month of August. From Glasgow cholera spread rapidly along the Clyde, along the canal and down the Ayrshire coast.[20]

James Arthur and his assistants faced the unenviable task of making a working reality out of the elegant plans which the Central Board of Health had set out in the circulars of autumn 1831. The medical agents of London had to come to terms with the local prejudices and power structure. As soon as he arrived in Glasgow, James Arthur saw the Lord Provost, who was persuaded to send a letter seeking the co-operation of all the county Lord Lieutenants. Although anxious to get to Kirkintilloch, James Arthur was even more anxious to get the support of the Duke of Hamilton, and waited to see the Duke before visiting the infected area; 'some alarm being felt about the palace respecting contagion'.[21] In Kirkintilloch support was less reserved. The Lord Provost, a local mill-owner, took Arthur to his factory at Campsie, persuaded the workpeople to subscribe for a hospital on the premises and let the army doctor talk to them about the need for early treatment.[22] The influence of paternalistic capital was fully behind the health measures. Others were more cautious. The shopkeepers of Ballinstone complained that the London Board had spoilt their trade by including the words '. . .and vicinity' in the published cholera returns. Two local canal boat companies were contacted but refused to co-operate in measures of quarantine.[23]

When Simeon Bullen reported for duty on 29 February, Arthur sent him to Kilwinning, a small weaving township three miles inland from Irvine on the Ayrshire coast. Cholera had been brought by Flora Johnson, a collier's wife who had walked from Springbank in search of work and stayed with a friend at Doura, a small hamlet in the parish. When Bullen arrived he found Doura was a filthy little settlement of 108 people. They had taken no precautions. They had few blankets or other necessities, and their medical man, Dr Anderson, a man whose constitution had been weakened by service in India, was himself a victim of cholera. Bullen's efforts to help were sadly hampered,

> The excitement amongst the populace of Kilwinning was so great that Mr Bullen although ordered to reside there, has been obliged to remain in Irvine – the person in Kilwinning who had procured him a lodging was threatened to have his house pulled down – a similar feeling exists generally amongst the lower classes.

Bullen himself explained that 'the poor people seem to imagine that I am to bring the disease there.' His only ally in the township was Archibald Campbell, the minister of the parish, who warned him to stay in Irvine as Kilwinning had no police or magistrates, but eventually the minister found lodgings for Bullen in a farmhouse two miles from the township, and promised to use the pulpit to ask for the support of the 'respectable' people against 'ignorance'. The church was the only agent of social authority on which the medical visitor could place any reliance. The small weaving, mining and ironworks villages of the west of Scotland suffered many small but intense outbreaks in early 1832. Although not geographically isolated, these villages remained hostile to the outside influence of the Board of Health men. Old Monkland and Carron Iron Works were equally unwelcoming when Arthur's young assistants arrived there. James Arthur himself was insulted and threatened with assault when called to Helensburgh by the magistrates to inspect a body. Thurston Caton was no happier with his reception at Paisley,

> from a strong feeling of dislike to medical men and their medicines (displaying itself by the hooting and shying of stones at the one – and the rejection of the other)...[cases] are seldom discovered till the remedies are of little avail.

Arthur became more and more despondent about the local response to the medical profession, 'the conduct of the mob in this part of the world has disgusted the good with the cause, and the bad never were friendly to it.'[24]

James Arthur and his assistants did have some limited success. They provided some emergency medical assistance. Arthur himself was a source of advice and comfort for the harrassed local authorities of the west and central lowlands, and his persuasion did result in some minor improvements in medical provision. His correspondence was a constant stream of requests for regular reporting of cases and in return came requests for help. At the start he wrote to all the sheriffs, provosts and surgeons asking for accurate returns. He reprimanded the medical men of Glasgow for not reporting cases amongst their private fee-paying patients. He met the Sheriff of Dunbarton to discuss the state of Kilwinning. James Salom of the Irvine Board of Health was advised to take all precautions, especially over early burial. Woodside, Irvine and Falkirk were criticised for their hospital plans, or lack of them, and all made various excuses. Old Monkland was urged to remove all nuisances and Belfast was warned of the approach of the *Isabella,* which had reported a case whilst windbound off Dumbarton Rock. There was, he told MacLean, little time for research or investigation into the clinical history of the disease.[25]

Arthur got little satisfaction from the work he did in Scotland. In the middle of April he wrote bitterly to MacLean,

> I have served more than thirty years in the Army under difficulties and in times as eventful as has fallen to the lot of any medical officer, but I have never experienced any service so unpleasant as the present – what between the hazards of the disease – the dangers of a lawless mob, the numerous perplexing references, the laborious extent of the responsibilities and the unsatisfactory result of one's exertions, I am extremely fatigued with the concern.[26]

To add to his woes, his service ended with a squalid little dispute over expenses. From the start James Arthur had dropped hints that his travelling expenses were inadequate to deal with a spreading epidemic. He claimed that the regulations for expenses which applied to army officers would be ruinous. He needed a choice of transport, instead of being restricted to public transport, for he was liable to be called out at all times of the day and night. In any case he objected to having to travel in public transport in an infected district. He wanted hotel instead of lodging-house accommodation and wanted his postage paid for his contacts with the Central Board. Eventually he received the devastating reply which has depressed many agents of government, '. . .as the rate of pay and allowance for travelling has been defined by a Treasury Minute, the Board cannot deviate therefrom. . .'[27] The whole episode ended with Arthur's curt dismissal. On 25 April he was told that his services would not be required after 8 May, and he would be paid off with a month's salary. MacLean was defensive and apologetic. The Board had no power over money; that was the Treasury. In any case he expected the Central Board soon to be finished itself as there were only two to three cases a day in the London area. It was not clear what was the reason for the dismissal of the medical agents. The government may have found that it was an expensive exercise which was having little obvious result and decided to take advantage of a lull in the epidemic to dismiss the men and leave everything to the local boards. They may have run out of funds and been forced to economise or even have been so misinformed about the regions that they genuinely thought that the job had been done. At any event the end of April saw a change of policy and a reduction in the amount of central direction of anti-cholera measures.

III

By the time cholera arrived in London on 9 February the Central Board of Health had only partially completed their reflections on the flaws which winter had revealed in their advice and administrative plans. This arrival was not announced until 16 February when the Central Board published ten cases along the Thames in their regular bulletin.[28] The first three were at Rotherhithe: an unemployed seaman, a coal-dredger and a ship-scraper who had been working on a collier from Newcastle. There was little doubt that the infection had been brought along the east coast trade route which was dominated by these colliers. London reacted in much the same way as Sunderland and Newcastle. The District Board of Health at Rotherhithe met with Mr Skeggs in the chair. He told them that their object was to contradict the Whitehall statement. They heard reports from the parish surgeon, who was employed by the Board, at least by those who were Poor Law officials, and from two other local surgeons. All agreed that the area had never been as healthy as the last six months and that, after detailed enquiries, they could find no symptoms of cholera in the reported cases. By this time the three men were dead.[29] Hume gave the same assurance to the House of Commons, and Poulett-Thompson told worried MPs that the district inspectors and physicians were checking all reports, whilst Henry Hunt, radical and orator, asked gloomily if the ventilation of the Commons could be improved.[30] The Westminster Medical Society debated the matter and decided that even if cholera were in London, which they doubted, it was certainly not infectious.[31] Cholera took little notice of the democracy of the meeting and spread rapidly throughout March and April. In May cases declined, causing a wave of false optimism; then came the tremendous mortality of July and August, 1,363 and 1,198, and the slow fading of the disease into the cold of winter.[32]

IV

During the winter of 1831-2 the Central Board of Health saw the crumbling of those plans which had been so carefully researched over the summer and published in the three great circulars. They never overcame two basic deficiencies. They lacked adequate authority and they lacked adequate information, both factual and theoretical. The circulars recommended a wide range of measures, cleansing streets, whitewashing houses, removing nuisances, setting up hospitals and isolating suspects, but the weakness of this plan rapidly became apparent as letters from the localities arrived in the Central Board offices. John Fenwick of Newcastle wanted an order on the overseers of St Andrew's Parish for the removal of nuisances in front of the barracks. Stockton found they were 'virtually prohibited' from removing nuisances in the manner proposed in the government circular, nor could they stop, unload and disinfect the carriers' carts as they had planned.[33] The Central Board had not anticipated this problem, for earlier in the month they had constituted the Stockton Board for just this purpose.[34] In the London suburbs the secretary of the Brompton Board found that nuisance removal could only be enforced by presentment at the Sessions, every three months, fine 19s.8d., and then only if the name of the owner of the property were known. York tried to exclude vagrants, but found like other towns that a man only became a 'vagrant' in the eyes of the law after he had stayed one night in the town; little use for excluding infection. The only authority which the Privy Council could give to the local boards rested on the statute, 6 George IV, c.78, and that meant quarantine. The Central Board began to realise this and advised Southwark that it was no good inspecting the water supply as they had no power to take action. Thus an instinctive move in the right direction was curbed at the start by inadequate power. A long and sorry letter from Haddington showed just how ineffective the Central Board's plans could be. The Board went promptly into action in December, but needed immediate knowledge of cases in order to isolate them. The local doctors soon found that there were no penalties for not reporting cases, so they stopped making their daily reports. The nuisance removal provisions were less use in Scotland than England, for the orders were to be given to the overseers of the poor, who did not exist in Scotland. Distance from Whitehall only increased problems. Privy Council orders granting authority took longer to obtain and even the circulars were more difficult to get hold of.

The greatest of all these failures of legal authority was the lack of effective power to raise local finance. The east coast ports were first to complain. Their trade was stopped and they had no money. In London in January, both Mile End and St Mary-le-bone found they had no funds to operate with and Liverpool wrote uneasily that the church wardens were providing money for health measures in the knowledge that it could be challenged as illegal even if the vestry voted by a majority in support of their expenditure – in fact the vestry refused to vote any money. Financial difficulties were even greater in Scotland, for most areas had no regular means for raising an assessment in the manner of the English poor law.

As the epidemic gathered pace, the letter books of the Central Board show a constant anxiety for information. On 28 December they asked Haddington and Newcastle for the details and circumstances of the first cases. Two days later the Lord Provost of Edinburgh was asked for details of cases, and the names of the Board of Health. In January Gateshead was asked to keep a register of all cholera patients in the hospital, because of 'the importance to the interest of humanity that permanent sources of information as to the history and progress of cholera in this country may be established'. February's correspondence was filled with a perpetual nagging for reports of new cases.[35] Sunderland's experience demonstrated that the lack of early and accurate information destroyed any chance that existed of containing cholera. The Whitehall Board now realised that it was rapidly losing control of the situation, and floundered around desperately trying to get the accurate information which any executive body needs before it can take effective action.

These difficulties forced the government to go urgently to Parliament for more legal powers for the Privy Council. The government had received the winter reports with somewhat confused complacency, but as soon as cholera reached London they acted with great promptitude. On 14 February Lord Althorp told Parliament that the Cholera Bill he was introducing needed a rapid passage. The Privy Council wanted to issue a new set of orders and found they had no power to do so. The Act, when it had passed through Parliament a week or so later, enabled two Privy Councillors to make, renew or revoke rules and regulations for preventing contagion spreading, for providing relief for the sick and for speedy interment. The rules were to be enforced by JPs with fines of £1 to £5. The Privy Council was also enabled through a local justice of the peace to order the overseers or Guardians of the Poor to pay any necessary money to the local board of health for expenses 'reasonably and properly incurred'. The

Containment Fails

Poor Law authorities were to raise the money through the local rates in the usual way. Scotland had no regular poor rate system, and a separate Act was passed requiring the raising of the money by the same means as the police rate, or in areas and towns with no police force, the same means of assessment as was used for the 'conversion of statute labour' – in other words the rate used to finance road-making under various national and local statutes. Thus only a few weeks before the major epidemic broke out the government had managed to construct a system of financial supply for its local boards of health from such fragments of existing local government as it could find, and so enabled the local men at least to act confidently in the knowledge that they could pay for what they were doing. Despite the sense of imminent danger felt by the Commons, there were still complaints. Peel felt that the cost should be borne at national level because the worst-hit areas – often the poorest areas, added Henry Hunt – would bear the cost of measures designed to protect surrounding areas. This idea was brushed aside because of the fear that national money spent at local level would lead to wasteful spending. The Scots feared the introduction of a compulsory poor rate assessment which they had always resisted as wasteful and a temptation to idleness. They also resented the need to apply for power to the Privy Council which meant seven days delay for them.

The Privy Council immediately issued an order (6 March) enabling areas threatened by cholera to establish a local board of health which would be authorised to set up a cholera hospital, purchase blankets, beds and medicines and hire domestic and nursing help. The local board would ask the parish vestry for authority to do this, and if the vestry refused they were to come to the Privy Council for a special Order in Council. This concern for setting up hospitals showed the Central Board still basically contagionist in its approach to cholera. It was not until late in the day (20 July), when the epidemic was spreading rapidly, that an order was issued giving powers for effective cleansing. The properly constituted local boards were at last given power of entry to 'any dwelling house, hut or cabin', 'upon receiving a certificate in writing signed by two medical practitioners'. Hog-styes, slaughter-houses, lodging-houses and drains, ditches and cesspools were given special mention. The same order required the burial of the cholera dead within 24 hours, and gave the local boards power to acquire special cholera burial grounds. The steady trickle of Orders in Council under the Cholera Act, which were published in the *London Gazette,* indicate that the Privy Council used the Act effectively for two major reasons. First, for breaking deadlocks caused by out-of-date administrative structures.

The older cities of England, especially the cathedral cities, were hopelessly fragmented into many parishes, which were the units of local Poor Law government. The Boards of Health were formed on a city basis, but faced the prospect of applying to over a dozen different groups of overseers for their cash, and the subsequent wrangles over apportionment. In Chester, Lincoln and Exeter, the Board was authorised to apply to the Guardians of the Poor, normally a money-spending authority looking after the workhouse, rather than a money-raising authority like the overseers. By far the largest number of orders were made to force reluctant overseers and vestries to pay up. This was done by way of a magistrate's order. Another minor class of orders provided a rapid way of solving minor legal difficulties such as the need to transfer a prisoner from the New Bailey prison in Manchester, or giving extra power to a local authority, as at Wednesbury and Bristol where the constable or magistrates were authorised to stop the holding of traditional fairs at the end of August and in Scotland where the justiciary were allowed to postpone their autumn circuit.[36] The Cholera Act brought a small addition to the authority of the Privy Council but did little to halt the spread of the epidemic. The situation rapidly got out of control. The decline of the epidemic was only brought about by the natural effect of winter cold. For most people that was the end of the epidemic. There were a few scattered outbreaks in 1833, notably during August in London, and there was one ferocious and isolated outbreak at Beith in Ayrshire, a place which had escaped in 1831-2. In December the Central Board of Health was dissolved. The Privy Council clerks kept the letter books open to deal with isolated outbreaks and administrative squabbles (mainly about cash), and cholera moved on to Ireland and the United States.

V

There is little to be gained by following the cholera, case by case, epidemic by epidemic, through the towns and villages of Britain.[37] Cholera's ability to reveal the quality and nature of British society must now be exploited. The first chapters have posed the problem which that society faced in 1832 and have shown the efforts and failures of the administration to deal with this threat. There were failures of authority, failures of information and failures of knowledge.

The approach and the incidence of cholera revealed the different interests, values, perspectives and resources of different social and economic groups in two ways, firstly in the choice of victims, and then

Table 3: Month by Month Progress of Cholera, 1831-1832

		Britain (excluding London)		London	
Year	Month	New Cases	Deaths	New Cases	Deaths
1831	Nov.	319	97	–	–
	Dec.	697	282	–	–
1832	Jan.	2,149	614	–	–
	Feb.	2,332	627	130	81
	Mar.	1,589	685	1,599	834
	Apr.	1,890	975	818	426
	May	1,575	678	125	70
	June	3,274	1,183	305	180
	July	9,135	3,454	3,027	1,362
	Aug.	20,912	7,635	2,939	1,240
	Sept.	11,269	4,794	1,347	685
	Oct.	8,575	3,698	700	382
	Nov.	2,139	789	27	13
	Dec.	325	138	3	2

Source: Sir David Barry, 'On the Statistics of Epidemic Cholera', *Transactions of the Statistical Society of London,* vol. 1, Part 1, 1837.

in the different reactions of different social groups to the threat and presence of epidemic. These must be examined over the whole range of society. The reactions of two specialised groups were important — the medical profession and the protagonists of various religious viewpoints.

Notes

1. Return of Pay and Allowances due to the undermentioned medical officers and civil medical gentlemen employed under the directions of the Central Board of Health up to the 8th June 1832..., and Monthly totals for medical gentlemen under the Board, P.R.O., P.C.1/110.
2. Rough Minutes of the Central Board of Health, 16 November 1831, P.R.O., P.C.1/105.
3. Cholera handbill, 29 October 1831, in the Wilson Collection vol.3, f.751, Newcastle upon Tyne Central Library; *Lancet,* 4 February 1832, p.672.
4. Two handbills, 10 and 15 November 1831, from vol.3 fol.755 and 756 of Wilson Collection; Letter from A. Reed, Mayor of Newcastle in the Rough Minutes of the Central Board of Health, 17 November 1831, P.R.O., P.C.1/105.

5. Letter from A. Reed, Mayor of Newcastle in the Rough Minutes of the Central Board of Health, 29 November 1831, P.R.O., P.C.1/105; Cholera Return in Great Britain, P.R.O., P.C.1/108; *The Courier*, 30 November to 10 December 1831.
6. *The Courier*, 10 to 24 December 1831; Cholera Return in Great Britain, loc. cit.
7. *Lancet*, 4 February 1832, p.672.
8. Dr David Craigie, 'Account of the Epidemic Cholera at Newburn in January and February 1832', *E.M.S.J.*, vol.37, 1832, pp.337-84; John Snow, *On the mode of communication of Cholera*, 2nd edition, London, 1855.
9. Letter from Mr Claxton, 5 New Bridge St., Newcastle, 8 January 1832, P.R.O., P.C.1/103.
10. Reports from Creagh on the Rough Minutes of the Central Board of Health, 21 to 29 December 1831, P.R.O., P.C.1/105.
11. Two letters from James Gibson Esq., Newcastle upon Tyne, 21 December 1831, P.R.O., P.C.1/103.
12. *Edinburgh Evening Courant*, 29 December 1831.
13. Letters from Major MacDonald to the Central Board of Health, Royal Hotel. Edinburgh, 28 December 1831, and 5 January 1832 and enclosures, P.R.O., P.C.1/107; *Edinburgh Evening Courant*, 29 and 31 December 1831.
14. *Edinburgh Evening Courant*, 21 January 1832.
15. *Lancet*, 4 February 1831, p.674; Dr Craigie, 'On the History and Etiology of Cholera', *E.M.S.J.*, vol.39, 1833, p.363.
16. James Y. Simpson, 'On the evidence of the occasional contagious propagation of malignant cholera', *E.M.S.J.*, vol.49, 1838.
17. *Cholera Gazette*, 14 February 1832.
18. Ibid.
19. James Y. Simpson, *E.M.S.J.*, vol.49, 1838.
20. Stewart to Arthur, 2 February 1832, P.R.O., P.C.1/107; George Watt, 'On the Origin and Spread of Cholera in Glasgow and its neighbourhood', *Glasgow Medical Journal*, vol.5, 1832, pp.298-394; James Cleland and James Corkindale, 'Conspectus of Cholera in Glasgow', *E.M.S.J.*, vol.39, 1833, pp.503-4.
21. Arthur to MacLean, Glasgow, 10 and 11 February 1832, P.R.O., P.C.1/107.
22. *Idem*, 11 February 1832.
23. Arthur to MacLean, 16 and 23 March 1832; Andrew Ranken, Monkland Canal Company Office to Arthur, 20 March 1832, and Arthur to MacLean, 13 February 1832, P.R.O., P.C.1/107.
24. Letters from Arthur to MacLean between 29 February and 28 March 1832, from Thurston Caton at Paisley to Arthur, 20 February 1832, from Simeon Bullen at Irvine to Arthur, 2 and 4 March 1832, from Archibald Campbell, The Manse, Kilwinning to Arthur, 4 March 1832, P.R.O., P.C.1/107.
25. From Dr Arthur's Correspondence Scotland, P.R.O., P.C.1/107.
26. Arthur to MacLean, 16 February 1832, P.R.O., P.C.1/107.
27. Arthur to MacLean, 10 March 1832, P.R.O., P.C.1/107.
28. *Lancet*, 18 February 1832.
29. *The Courier*, 16 February 1832.
30. *Hansard's Parliamentary Debates*, vol.10, 13 February and 5 March 1832.
31. *The Courier*, 20 February 1832.
32. *Reports on the Epidemic Cholera...*, William Baly and William W. Gull, London, 1854, p.30.
33. *Papers relating to cholera*, P.P. (H. of C.) 1831-32, XXVI.
34. Central Board of Health letter book, 9 December 1832, P.R.O., P.C.1/93.
35. *Papers relating to cholera*, P.P. 1831-32, XXVI; Central Board of Health letter book, December 1832 to February 1832, P.R.O., P.C.1/93.
36. The information about the Privy Council was taken from the *London Gazette*,

1832, *passim*, and that on the Cholera Act debates from *Hansard's Parliamentary Debates*, 3rd series, vol.10, 1832.
37. See Charles Creighton, *A history of epidemics*, vol.2, London, 1891, pp.793-862; N. Longmate, *King Cholera*, London, 1966.

5 VICTIMS

Cholera killed some 32,000 people in Britain in 1831 and 1832. Of most of these people, no more was recorded than where and when they died. For some the local Board of Health Minute Book or a well-kept parish register contain a brief outline of the manner of their death and their state in life: 174 entries were carefully written into the records of the Oxford Board of Health.

> James Bristow, age 26, residence, Castle Gaol of Oxford, Criminal Prisoner in the Castle Gaol, seized 24 June at 10 p.m., died 25 June at 4 p.m., buried in the Castle, his surgeon was Mr J.F. Wood.
>
> John Watts, age 42, he lodged at the Shoulder of Mutton in St Thomas's; his condition of life, a travelling mendicant drawn by four dogs, seized 30 June at 3 p.m., died 3 July at 11 a.m., buried in St Thomas's, his surgeon was Mr John Symonds.
>
> James Wright, age 35 of St Thomas's, a labourer, seized 6 July and died 8 July, buried in St Ebbe's, treated by Mr Dickeson.
>
> Adam Henderson Bowell, age 2¼, of Godfrey's Row, St Ebbe's, condition of life simply recorded as 'labourer', seized and died on the 6 July and buried in St Ebbe's.
>
> Elizabeth Bowell, age 11 months, again condition of life 'labourer', seized 7 July, died 7 July, buried St Ebbe's.

These short chronicles were followed by others, some children, some prisoners and mendicants on the fringes of society, most were labourers, craftsmen, or their wives.[1]

The parish register of Leith in the County of Edinburgh was even more sparing in detail.

> John Jack, tidesman, age 60, buried 1st May at 5 a.m., died 29 April.
>
> Philadelphia Fotheringham, relict of tidesman, age 57, buried 2 May at 6 a.m., died on the 1st.
>
> John Hercules, labourer, buried 12 May at 5 a.m., having died on the 10th.

These men and women were hurried to their graves at dawn by the anxious and fearful authorities of Leith.[2]

The letters, returns and post-mortem reports of the correspondents of the Central Board of Health contain brief portraits of victims, where death and official attention has recorded the end of a life that otherwise would have attracted little notice. Most were wage-earners, labourers and craftsmen, like Rodenbury, 'the industrious shoemaker' of Sunderland who 'dined and supped on Pork, drank no fermented liquor, and went to bed well'. He awoke with terrifying vomiting and purging which 'filled several chamber pots' and was dead by afternoon.[3] Others came from the fringes of society. They did not even have that claim on the national product which selling their labour might command. John Solomon, Providence Court, White's Yard, Rosemary Lane, a member of London's poor Jewish community, made his living picking coal and wood from the waterside until he died of cholera aged 50. In Newcastle, Ann Dennison died in December 1831; she 'has been debauched for some time and had an abortion a fortnight ago'.[4] A prostitute from the Nungate was among the first to die in Haddington. She was a drunkard, blind and addicted to narcotics. Cholera also found many passive patient victims waiting in the poverty into which unemployment and casual labour had brought them. In late November, Dr Barry found two daughters in the cholera hospital at Sunderland. The mother and the other two children were sick at home, with no food, the one blanket given them two days before, and another child dead.[5]

Not all victims came from the poor and working classes. Glasgow especially had been worried by its middle-class cases. At Rothesay, the first case was a 'respectable' person in 'comfortable circumstances' who lived by the Bridge, followed by the death of an old doctor, Dr Fyfe, but 'he was very intemperate and irregular in his habits'.[6] The case of Mrs Haslewood, the wife of the Sunderland surgeon, showed the fortunes of a middle-class victim. She had attended the post-mortem of Rodenbury and Sproat on 1 November. She was, her husband reported, age 28 and in perfect health. She was seized at church with dreadful pains in the stomach, and carried home to a warm bed, where she was subjected to bleeding, opium and brandy followed by rhubarb and magnesia with beef tea and negus when the spasms ceased. Negus was a comforting drink of wine, warmed before the fire, and mixed with boiling water and lemon, with nutmeg and sugar to taste. Mrs Haslewood was then carefully nursed back to health. The rest of the family, including the baby, nine months old, remained well and sent their thanks to Dr Daun for his 'kindness and attention' in looking after Mrs Haslewood. The middle class was able to provide extra comfort and attention which

Victims

scarcely concealed the pain of the disease or the haphazard, often savage nature, of the treatment offered.[7]

There are few sources of objective information about the epidemic which indicate whether these sketches and portraits were typical of the 32,000 dead. The most complete records were made by the Central Board. Form 5, 'General Statistical Return' was sent out to local boards with each circular. The information on this form was collated by Sir William Pym at the end of the epidemic. He constructed a map which was deposited in the Royal Library at the wish of the King, though it no longer appears to be in that library. He also made a voluminous table or index, 'Cholera Returns in Great Britain', a copy of which is still in the Privy Council papers.[8]

A few places did collect detailed statistics in a systematic manner. The initial question is a somewhat surprising one; was anyone in a real sense a victim of cholera? Did cholera cause extra deaths or just replace other, perhaps less painful, causes of death in the dangerous urban environments of 1832? At the time many claimed that cholera did not raise the death rate and observed that apart from cholera, 1832 was an exceptionally healthy period.[9] The claim that cholera was a replacement cause of death rather than an extra cause of death is a difficult one to test because of the lack of firm national figures for cholera, and the lack of any overall figures at all for death rates. There was local evidence. Both Robert Cowan in Glasgow and James Stark in Edinburgh used the parish registers to provide information on the total deaths within the two cities, so that the figures are burial rates rather than true death rates. Cowan certainly included the burial of still-born children in his totals and these represent something like 2 per thousand in the burial rates given in Table 4. Stark's figures were consistently lower, suggesting that Edinburgh was the healthier city. This may have been true, but direct comparison between the cities is unwise on these figures, for Stark may well have excluded still-born burials and have been less thorough in his survey of the registers. Comparison between years within the same city is valid and shows clearly that cholera caused an increase in deaths and that there was no compensating fall in death rate after 1832. The rates rarely fell back to those of the 1820s and indeed in the typhus year of 1837 the death rate again approached that of 1832.

Cholera not only added to deaths but also selected its victims from the age groups in a manner different from the normal causes of death. Cleland's careful statistical work provided the age structure of Glasgow's population in 1831, which the official census does not, and age-specific

Table 4: Burial Rates in Glasgow and Edinburgh, 1827-1837

	Glasgow*		Edinburgh	
Population 1831	202,420		139,123	
Cholera Deaths 1832	3,174		1,159	
Year	Burials	Crude Burial Rate	Burials	Crude Burial Rate
1827	5,136	28.5	3,347	25.9
1828	5,942	32.0	3,696	28.1
1829	5,452	28.5	3,164	23.6
1830	5,185	26.3	3,510	25.7
1831	6,547	32.3	3,664	26.3
1832	10,278	49.0	5,262	37.8
1833	6,632	30.6	4,312	30.9
1834	6,728	30.0	3,657	26.2
1835	7,849	34.0	3,543	25.4
1836	9,143	38.3	3,968	28.4
1837	10,886	44.3	5,009	35.8

*Data for Glasgow included the Gorbals and Barony areas.

Source: Robert Cowan, *Vital Statistics of Glasgow. . .*, Glasgow, 1838, pp.7 and 10; James Stark, *Inquiry into some points of the Sanitary State of Edinburgh. . .*, Edinburgh, 1847, p.11.

burial figures for 1830 and 1832, including overall totals and cholera figures. These figures have been converted into age-specific burial rates (Table 5). The pattern of death in a normal year had two characteristic features. There were massive casualties among children under five. The rate was even higher among the youngest of this group. Once past the age of five, life became relatively safer until the fifties age group, when deaths again rose above the average. The cholera pattern was different. Children were relatively safe, teenagers even safer. For adults the chance of death from cholera rose much more rapidly than the risk of death from other causes. Thus the 'extra' deaths which were caused by cholera were principally among the middle-aged. The bulk of the normal death toll consisted of young children. Whilst it would be wrong to underestimate the suffering and sadness left in the vast majority of families by child deaths, these deaths nevertheless did the minimum of social and economic damage to the family, if only because most families were organised to produce large numbers of children, and so ensure that

Victims 83

some remained to reach adulthood. Cholera added to deaths among age groups for which the family had no such compensation. Many victims had families dependent on them for economic and emotional support. When they died, the widows and orphans were left as an extra charge on the Poor Law, and the children suffered all the disruption of a broken home, not by the breakdown of marriage, but by premature death.

Table 5: Impact of Cholera on the Population of Glasgow, 1832: Age Structure

Age In years	Population 1831[a]	Burials 1830[b]	Age-specific Burial[c] Rates per 1000 1830	Cholera Burials[d] 1832	Age-specific Burial[e] Rates per 1000 from Cholera in 1832
Under 5	30,277	2,000	66.06	130	4.29
5-10	25,707	253	9.84	106	4.12
10-20	41,956	276	6.57	132	3.14
20-30	38,185	334	8.74	358	9.37
30-40	26,419	313	11.84	529	20.02
40-50	18,014	348	19.31	639	35.47
50-60	11,648	352	30.21	556	47.73
60-70	6,920	339	48.98	444	64.16
Over 70	3,300	499	151.21	272	82.42
Total	202,426	5,185 (total includes 471 still-born)	25.61	3,166	15.64

Sources:
 a. and b., J. Cleland, *Ennumeration of the Inhabitants of the City of Glasgow...*, Glasgow, 1832, p.11.
 c. Calculated from a. and b. Hence liable to be underestimated.
 d. J. Cleland and J. Carbindale, 'Conspectus of Cholera in Glasgow...', *E.M.S.J.*, vol.39, 1833, pp.500-6.
 e. Calculated from a. and d., hence liable to be overestimated.

Since the cholera first appeared in Moscow major interest has always focused on the social status and the social class of the victims. As the cholera crossed Europe, the periodicals gave a comforting image of the cholera victim. In Hamburg, cholera had been confined to beggars and vagrants and after the initial alarm, parties and amusements had continued as normal, was the report from the *Monthly Review*. Its competitor for the general literary drawing room readers claimed, 'it will be and hitherto has been confined to the poor, the distressed, the badly fed, the badly clothed, the filthy and the intemperate.' Once the poverty theory of cholera had been accepted, protection for the individual was simple, 'A broad cloth without and a warm heart within will be entire surities against the invasion of cholera to any hurtful degree.' The 'more respectable and prosperous sections of society' felt sure that they would be safe from cholera.[10]

The closer examination of European evidence made by the medical journals did not justify this confidence. The *Edinburgh Medical and Surgical Journal* agreed that the majority of victims were from the lower classes but warned that this might be no more than their due proportion in populations of which they formed the vast majority. When information was available on the deaths in different social classes, the picture was not so simple. In Moscow at least 11.5 per cent of the 4,588 deaths which had occurred by 20 January 1831 came from the better ranks, the nobility, gentry, superior military officers, magistrates, clergy and merchants. This was about the same proportion as their share in the total population. After looking at the Berlin *Cholera Gazette* the *Journal* concluded that 10 per cent of the thousand people attacked before 15 October were from the class of professional men, schoolmasters, artists, merchants, manufacturers and people of independent fortune, though the better classes were increased by the addition of 28 underclerks. This 10 per cent nearly equalled the proportion the higher classes bore in the total population. In Warsaw some 4.8 per cent of the cases were from the 'better ranks', well below their share in total population. The *Journal* drew from this an analysis that was as relevant for Britain as for Europe. In Moscow and Berlin the houses of noblemen and merchants were intermingled with those of their servants and others from lower social classes. In Warsaw, the dwellings of different classes were more segregated. The rich lived in one quarter and thus largely escaped cholera.[11] The relative geographical segregation of social classes was a key factor in differentiating the life chances of the classes in the face of cholera.

When cholera arrived in Britain, the newspapers and the reports of many medical men gave the same impression. Samuel Smith and William Hey, both physicians, visited north-east England and returned to tell a meeting at Leeds that only three 'respectable' people had been attacked in Newcastle and the rest were of 'the lowest class, living in crowded apartments and addicted to habits of intemperance'. Henry Dodd, the surgeon at Houghton-le-Spring, claimed that cholera was 'the poor man's disease'. In the spring the impressions of London were much the same. Francis MacCann wrote to the *Courier* in February to say that cholera did not affect 'the more respectable classes of society'.[12] Another letter to the *Standard* gave a fairly balanced selection of the case histories being presented to the public:

Florence Sullivan, brewer's vat maker,
 '...a small but not uncomfortable room' where the body was laid out for a week according to Irish custom (Southwark)'
Francis Byrne,
 '...this poor boy, whose state was most wretched'
another victim from
 'Vine Street; a miserable filthy court, consisting of small thickly inhabited wooden houses'.
The reports from the north were much the same,
 '...an elderly female, a collector of old clothes',
who died in the Canongate, Edinburgh; the first victims in Glasgow,
 '...an old man in very poor circumstances',
and Janet Lindsay,
 'an old woman very much addicted to whiskey'.[13]

It was not a picture of filth and poverty all the way, but those qualities so dominated the reports that it must have been easy for the respectable middle-class business-owner, professional man or tradesman to say, 'Cholera is not a threat to me.' It was easy for *The Times* to say, 'The real causes of the disease are poverty, bad living, insufficient clothing, dirty streets and dwellings, united with occasional excess.'[14]

Cobbett, who had used his pen to educate and reflect the thoughts of his working-class readers for over a decade, might mock the implication that his readers were filthy, drunken and frequenters of stinking brothels, but there was little that he or anyone else could do to break the comforting image of the victim as lower-class, filthy, poor and drunken.[15]

This image was the dominant middle- and upper-class perception of the cholera victims. Quite a different view was offered by James Kay, physician to the Ardwick and Ancoates Dispensary and Secretary to the Manchester and district Board of Health, when he wrote *The Moral and Physical Conditions of the Working Classes* to draw the attention of the wealthier, rate-paying, charitable subscribing portions of Manchester to the lesson which he felt cholera should have taught them. Before the epidemic, claimed Kay, the prosperous capital-owning, manufacturing, trading and professional people of Manchester had well understood the lower and working classes as a threat of riot, crime, political and trades union challenge, now they understood them as a threat of disease,

> The ingress of a disease, which threatens, with a stealthy step, to invade the sanctity of the domestic circle; which may be unconsciously conveyed from those haunts of beggary where it is rife into the most still and secluded retreat of refinement – whose entrance, wealth cannot absolutely bar, and luxury invites, this is an event. . .which ensures that the anxious attention of every order of society shall be directed to that in which social ills abound.[16]

As a result, predicted Kay, the wealthier classes would now seek to improve the moral and material conditions of the working classes in order to secure 'their personal safety'. Although Kay's view has impressed many historians, it was a minority perception of the epidemic. It does, however, presage developments later in the century, when middle-class fear of cholera spreading from the lower classes became a real factor in reform, and it does reflect the underlying reality of the biological basis of class revealed by cholera a little better than the majority view.

Both Kay and the majority view assumed that society was divided into two social groups, a respectable upper and middle class who were responsible, comparatively safe and held all rightful sources of power, and a lower class who were addicted to drink, poor, dangerous, and in general victims of cholera. Cholera consciousness was a consciousness of two nations on the Disraelian pattern. The two-nation model of society, the division between the rich and the poor, those with power and those without power, those responsible for taking action against cholera and those threatened by cholera, was only one contemporary perception of British society. It simplified and obscured reality. The power division altered according to the perspective of the observer. At national level, Lord Londonderry and Lord Melbourne, with their land and political authority, John Marshall with his industrial capital and county estates, Charles Greville with the authority of the Privy Council, stood apart as policy and regulation-makers who dominated the surgeons, shopkeepers and ships' captains of the cholera areas. At local level, the petty autocrats of the Poor Law Overseer's office, the parish surgeon, the chairman of the committee collecting subscriptions for the poor, the ratepayers and owners of petty capital all held power to protect or neglect the fortunes of those who had little more power than the ability to sell their labour when the market gave them the opportunity.

Nor did wealth and income or social status give a clear division into rich and poor; instead there was an infinite gradation of economic well-being and social prestige, which was recognised by contemporaries in their reference to middle classes and labouring classes, plural. In Cleland's Glasgow wages ranged from 3s.3d. per day for sawyers, through 2s.4d. for the masons to 1s.6d. for their labourers and less for the unfortunate hand loom weavers, whilst the paupers in the Town's Hospital only had £5 to £10 a year spent on each of them. Income and status was influenced by birth, by type of job and by property owned. The minister of the kirk in Glasgow who only earned £425 might gain as much prestige as the merchant who took several thousand a year from his business. The Leeds flax spinner John Marshall had used some of the profits from his mill to buy huge estates in the Lake district but would stand equal in prestige with men of less property but aristocratic birth.[17]

Occupational divisions and inequalities of property, prestige and power created differences in life style, in opportunities and expectations which were and are the basis of class distinction. Inequality among classes was not just a matter of income, housing and education, but a matter of life itself. The figures produced by Chadwick when he made his great report on the health of the labouring classes in 1842, as well as local studies like that made by Robert Stark in Edinburgh in 1847, all showed that the lower and working classes lost more children in infancy and died earlier if they reached adult life.[18] Though most observers were confident that this situation obtained in the cholera epidemic of 1832, Kay was not so sure.

Before the Registrar-General began his work in 1839 there was no regular recording of deaths, and the records which were made in chapel and parish registers rarely gave cause of death and occupation with any consistency or confidence, but the varied reactions to cholera produced a few records which provide brief glimpses of the relationship between cholera and occupation and status. They enable the historian to outflank the stereotyped view of middle-class newspapers and periodicals which, though perfect evidence of the nature of middle-class perception, act as an almost impenetrable barrier between historians and fact. In order to generalise about the status of the victims of cholera and compare them with the population as a whole, they have been placed by occupation in four status groups:

Class I: gentry and professional people

Class II: merchants, shopkeepers, master tradesmen and clerks
Class III: artisans, labourers and servants
Class IV: paupers and vagrants
Class V: a residual of those whose occupations were not given

In their history of the Sunderland epidemic Haslewood and Mordey gave the occupations of many of the first 64 cases. Similar information came from information sent to the Privy Council on the Newburn epidemic (2 January to 4 February 1832), Gaulter's study of Manchester (first 200 cases), and the records of the Oxford Board of Health.

Table 6: The First 64 Cases in Sunderland

I	*Gentry and Professional*	3
	Surgeon 3	
II	*Tradesmen and Clerks*	4
	Pilot, Tidewaiters 4	
III	*Artisans and Labourers*	43
	Shoemaker, Joiner, Tailor, Hatter 7	
	Keelman 14	
	Sailor 4	
	Nurse 2	
	Prostitute 5	
	Gardener, Washerwoman, Fisherwoman 4	
	Others 7	
IV	*Paupers*	5
V	*Unknown*	9
	TOTAL	64

Source: W. Haslewood and W. Mordey, *The History and Medical Treatment of Cholera as it appeared in Sunderland in 1831,* London, 1832.

Victims 89

Table 7: Newburn: Those who Died between 2 January and 4 February 1832

I	*Gentry and Professional*	2
	The Vicar and the Surgeon's Wife 2	
II	*Tradesmen and Clerks*	1
	Publican 1	
III	*Artisans and Labourers*	17
	Butcher, Dressmaker, 2	
	Fisherman and Waterman 2	
	Colliers and Miners 8	
	Labourers 4	
	Nurse 1	
IV	*Paupers*	10
V	*Unknown*	26
	TOTAL	56

Source: P.C.1/111.

Table 8: Manchester: The First 200 Cases

I	*Gentry and Professional*	1
	Surgeon 1	
II	*Tradesmen and Clerks*	17
	Rent Collector 2	
	Schoolmaster 1	
	Shopkeepers and Dealers 14	
III	*Artisans and Labourers*	144
	Textile Workers 75	
	(of which weavers 28 and spinners 8)	
	Skilled Trades 41	
	(of which sawyers and joiners 8, cobblers 11)	
	Unskilled 28	
IV	*Vagrant and Casual*	18
V	*Unknown*	20
	TOTAL	200

Source: Henry Gaulter, *The Origins and Progress of the Malignant Cholera in Manchester...*, London, 1833.

Table 9: Oxford: 174 Cases

I	*Gentry and Professional*	2
	At College 1	
	Gentleman 1	
II	*Tradesmen and Clerks*	11
	Bookseller 2	
	Innkeeper, Property in houses, Schoolkeeper 3	
	Sexton 1	
	Fishmonger, Greengrocer, Butcher, Shopkeeper 4	
	Musician 1	
III	*Artisans and Labourers*	109
	Skilled 21	
	(Of which engravers 3, boat-builders 2, printers 3, stone-masons 5)	
	Carpenter, Sawyer, Printer, Shoemaker 24	
	Clothes and Furnishing 10	
	(Of which tailors 3)	
	Transport 5	
	Labourers and Servants 30	
	Police and Soldiers 7	
	Nurses 2	
	Others 10	
IV	*Paupers* (including those in prison)	17
V	*Unknown*	35
	TOTAL	174

Source: 'Tabular View of the Cases of Cholera Morbus', produced by the Oxford Board of Health, Bodleian Library, Oxford.

Victims   91

These tables may be summarised in the following way. The first figure in each column is the number of cases or deaths. The figure in brackets represents cases or deaths as a percentage of the total with known occupations.

Table 10: Cholera and Occupational Status 1831-1832

(a)

Status	Sunderland	Newburn	Manchester	Oxford
I	3 (5.5)	2 (6.7)	1 (0.6)	2 (1.4)
II	4 (7.8)	1 (3.3)	17 (9.4)	11 (7.9)
III	43 (78.2)	17 (56.6)	144 (78.4)	109 (78.4)
IV	5 (9.1)	10 (33.3)	18 (12.23)	17 (12.2)
Total	55	30	180	139

The fluctuations within each category are considerable. This arises from the small numbers involved in I and II, and from the different proportions of paupers in each group. It was not clear if this was a real difference or if it represented the differing willingness to label or be labelled as a pauper or as a member of the occupation which had left the individual destitute. If the middle-class groups and the labouring-class groups are merged a clearer pattern emerges.

(b)

Status	Sunderland	Newburn	Manchester	Oxford
I and II	7 (12.7)	3 (10.0)	18 (10.0)	13 (9.3)
III and IV	48 (87.3)	27 (90.0)	162 (90.0)	126 (90.7)

Thus, in four places of very different social and economic structure, the east coast port, the mining village, the merchanting and manufacturing centre of cotton textiles, and the county and university town, the middle class made up 10 per cent of the victims of cholera and the working classes 90 per cent. This conclusion needs qualification. It is representative of urban victims but not of the rural areas, for the village of Newburn was exceptional in many ways. It was a mining rather than agricultural centre and suffered an explosive epidemic, not the few isolated cases which were more typical of the rural areas.

Table 10 (b) shows clearly that more working-class people were victims of cholera than middle-class people, which is not surprising given the numerical superiority of the working classes in British society.

Still, taking occupation as an indicator of status, 10 per cent of the victims in the four groups studied came from the middle classes. If these classes were not as safe from cholera as they thought were they comparatively safe in the manner which Chadwick's figures were to suggest they were from other diseases? An indirect estimate of their comparative safety in Manchester and Sunderland may be made using the poll books and the printed returns of the 1831 census, and assuming that those who voted on the new £10 franchise were from the middle class as Parliament had indeed intended.

Table 11: Cholera and Status in Sunderland and Manchester

	Sunderland			Manchester		
	Dead		Total	Dead		Total
Classes I and II	7	in	5,248	18	in	40,463
Classes III and IV	48	in	37,830	162	in	146,539
	Chances of appearing in the first					
	64 cases			200 cases		
Classes I and II	1	in	785	1	in	2,248
Classes III and IV	1	in	783	1	in	904

These figures do not give absolute values for the chances of catching cholera in each social class in each town, but they do have a comparative value within each town. Tables 10 and 11 need some qualification and interpretation. The 'unknowns' who have been left out of the calculation might properly have been added to the lower classes, as it seems inherently more likely that those with low social status should have had occupations which the investigators could not ascertain from directories, friends or neighbours. In the upper classes those whose occupation was unknown were called 'gentlemen'. Thus there is a likely underestimate of working-class victims. On the other hand several of the tradesmen, carpenters, printers, hatters, etc., who have been included in Class III may have been masters and should have been included in Class II, thus balancing the relative losses to the working classes through 'unknowns'.

The scant evidence which is available suggests that middle-class victims tended to come later in an epidemic after water supplies had become infected or the disease had been brought from the poorer

Victims 93

districts by servants. The early parts of epidemics predominate in these figures. The majority of the middle-class deaths recorded here came from specialised groups. Four out of eight deaths in Class I were surgeons (five if the surgeon's wife in Newburn is included). Several of those in Class II had occupations which would involve considerable contact with the lower classes, rent-collector, schoolmaster and tide-waiter. Others, like the shopkeepers and dealers of Manchester, may have been from small businesses living on credit and their own sweated labour and serving the working-class districts from which the other victims came.

In Manchester rents were high so that many wage-earners gained the £10 franchise. Thus the differential calculated would be wider than it should be; still, it seems likely that the increased geographical segregation of social classes, made possible by the greater size, wealth and rate of expansion of Manchester had increased the comparative safety of the middle classes.

Even if some of the assumptions made in these calculations are wrong, it is unlikely that the recalculated results would agree with the impression of safety which the middle class gained from their news media. The willingness of the middle and upper classes to identify cholera with the poor can partly be explained by wishful thinking, but also by the distribution of cholera within the middle class. Apart from the medical men it affected the lower ranks of the middle class, so that the more prominent members of the class, merchants, manufacturers and solicitors, escaped, increasing the general sense of false security which had been created by moral assumptions and impressionistic reporting. All detailed studies of middle-class behaviour in the epidemic suggest that this sense of security predominated, and that James Kay's belief that middle-class fear of cholera spreading from the working classes was an active element in class relationships during the epidemic, leading to help for the lower classes and perhaps later public health reform, was not justified.

Notes

1. 'Synopsis of Cases, Oxford, 1832', MSS Top Oxon c.303, Bodleian Library, Oxford.
2. Parochial Register of Leith, 1820-42, West Register House, Edinburgh, 692/15.
3. Post-Mortem Report from W. Haslewood, Sunderland, 1 November 1831.
4. Post-Mortem Reports, February 1832, P.R.O., P.C.1/103; Report from R. Glanton, Newcastle-upon-Tyne, 14 December 1831, P.R.O., P.C.1/103.
5. Dr Barry, Sunderland, 22 November 1831, P.R.O., P.C.1/105.
6. Thomas MacLauchlan, M.D., Rothesay, 15 April 1832, P.R.O., P.C.1/107.

94 *Cholera 1832*

7. W. Haslewood, Sunderland, 11 November 1831, P.R.O., P.C.1/103; for negus see, as ever, Mrs Isabella Beeton, *The Book of Household Management*. My edition is 1888, see p.943.
8. 'Cholera Returns of Great Britain', P.R.O., P.C.1/108; Sir David Barry, 'On the Statistics of Epidemic Cholera', *Transactions of the Statistical Society of London*, vol.1, Part 1, 1837.
9. *E.M.S.J.*, vol.69, 1848, p.382.
10. *The Monthly Review*, 1831, vol.3, n.s., p.450; *New Monthly Magazine*, vol.34, 1832, p.277; *The British Critic*, vol.11, 1832, p.376.
11. *E.M.S.J.*, vol.37, 1832, pp.190-4.
12. *Lancet*, 1832, p.798; cutting from the *Leeds Mercury* annotated by Dr MacCann, 'not enough evidence', P.R.O., P.C.1/103; *Courier*, 16 February 1832.
13. *Standard*, 22 February 1832; the letter had originally appeared in *The Times*.
14. *Times*, 13 February 1832; Mr West, 'The origin and spread of Cholera in Glasgow', *Glasgow Medical Journal*, vol.5, 1832.
15. *Cobbett's Political Register*, vol.74, 10 December 1831.
16. J.P. Kay, *The Moral and Physical Conditions of the Working Classes Employed in the Cotton Manufacture of Manchester*, Manchester, 1832, pp.11-12.
17. J. Cleland, *Statistical Tables Relative to Glasgow*, Glasgow, 1837; W.G. Rimmer, *Marshalls of Leeds, flax-spinners, 1788-1886*, Cambridge, 1960.
18. E. Chadwick, *Report on the Sanitary Condition of the Labouring Population of Great Britain*, edited with introduction by M.W. Flinn, Edinburgh, 1965, pp.220-3.

6 CLASS, POWER AND CHOLERA

The distribution of death indicated the relative safety of the upper and middle classes, with the exception of marginal groups and one specialised occupation. The perception of lower-class fortunes suggested imperfect knowledge despite superior resources. These were static aspects of class. Class relationships were more than this. They were based on the distribution of legitimate power; power over wealth, capital and resources, power over legitimate authority, the ability to control and influence the behaviour of others, power to defend property, life and deeply valued customs. The unequal distribution of such power was the basis of class. Conflict arose from the inequality itself, but the intensification of conflict usually arose when the expectations which one class held about the behaviour of others were disappointed. Conflicts and reactions during the cholera epidemic are best understood within the 'two nations' model. There were two other elements. Two groups of radicals provided an important link between the middle and working classes. The working-class radicals explained, modified and led the opinions of the working classes. Middle-class radicals challenged the traditional assumptions of their own class from within. The legitimate authority of the middle and upper classes was divided between the localities, where it was controlled by middle-class politicians and capitalists, and the national base where it was controlled by the ruling class and their aides. Conflicts between these two sorts of power foci played a crucial part in directing behaviour during the epidemic.

Cholera revealed class relationships in a number of ways. Each class reacted in a different way to the threat of cholera because their resources and past experience of disease were different. The tension caused by cholera also altered the behaviour of the classes towards each other. The middle and upper classes, who saw the speed and destructiveness of cholera as a threat to the health and economic and social stability of the society on which their privilege depended, reacted in a striking and unusual manner. From a working-class viewpoint this reaction was a threat to their normal life and legitimate rights far more serious than anything promised by cholera itself.

The bulk of the evidence we have on cholera came from administrative and middle-class sources, government, medical men, ministers of religion and a few middle-class biographies. There is little beyond our imagination to suggest what it felt like to watch and wait as cholera spread among cheap and crowded housing. The nearest the records come to the feelings of potential victims were occasional handbills and the radical press. These journals, Cobbett's long running *Political Register, Carpenter's Political Magazine,* John Doherty's *Poor Man's Advocate* and Henry Hetherington's *Poor Man's Guardian,* all reflected the feelings of their readers through the preoccupations of the political campaigns which attracted their authors — parliamentary reform, trades union interests and the repeal of the newspaper stamp duties.[1]

(i) Humbug

Through the distorting lenses of such evidence, the initial reaction of the poor and working classes was clear and can be summed up in one word — humbug. The point was made clearly in the broadsheet ballad printed by J.V. Quick of Clerkenwell and written for the tune of 'All people that on earth do dwell.'[2]

> All you that does in England dwell,
> I'll endeavour for to please you well,
> If you will listen, I will tell
> About the Cholera Morbus.
>
> In every street as you pass by,
> Take care they say or you will die,
> While others cry, 'It's all my eye',
> There is no Cholera Morbus.
>
> They say the doctors all went round,
> Through every part of London town,
> But it was no where to be found,
> It was off, the Cholera Morbus.
>
> Some people say it was a puff,
> It was done to raise the Doctor's stuff,
> And there has now been near enough,
> About the Cholera Morbus.

Cobbett noted with obvious approval a poster which had been placarded on the walls of Lambeth at the end of February,

CHOLERA HUMBUG! – Inhabitants of Lambeth, be not imposed upon by the villainously false reports that the Asiatic Cholera has reached London. A set of half-starved doctors, apothocaries' clerks, and jobbers in the parish funds, have endeavoured to frighten the nation into a lavish expenditure; with the Government they have succeeded in carrying a Bill which will afford fine pickings. A ruinous system of taxation, starvation, and intemperance, has been long carried on; it has now arrived at its acme, and disease is the natural result.[3]

In the early days of the Glasgow epidemic, James Arthur's insistence that local doctors should neither conceal nor neglect to report cases seemed a sensible attempt to increase the stream of accurate information coming to the administration. To the radical *Loyal Reformer's Gazette* the activities of a man paid £50 a month from public taxes were only an attempt to 'get up' cases to keep himself in a job. Dozens of ordinary deaths, the *Gazette* claimed, were being attributed to cholera by the doctors. There was the man whose daughter died of an ordinary bowel complaint, another whose child died of typhus, and the well-known case of Gruer M'Gruer who died from a burst blood vessel and was entered in the Board of Health books as 'real malignant cholera', when everyone knew that the real cause was 'dram drinking'.[4]

Past experience, epitomised in Paine's *Rights of Man,* and extended by the radical Press, had taught working-class radicalism that government was a corrupt organisation in the hands of the aristocracy who used their powers of taxation to create 'jobs' for themselves and their followers. Local government at town and parish level was equally adapted to providing corrupt profits for those less well endowed with statutory power – tradesmen and shopkeepers who ate the dinners and took the overpriced contracts paid for by rates that should have gone to help the poor. The lower strata of society had long experienced deception from government, professional men and tradesmen. When such a government warned them of cholera and began handing out 'jobs' to the medical men and orders to tradesmen, it was natural that the announcement was seen as yet another deception.

These views on government corruption were shared by a substantial portion of the middle class, whose views were represented in Parliament by a small but vocal army of MPs like Hume, Roebuck and Warburton. Middle-class radicalism added a touch of acid to *The Times* which provided approving corroboration of the radical picture of East London in February 1832:

The suspicion is very general throughout the City that the alarm has been spread through interested motives. The druggists' shops at all events, are already reaping the benefit of it. Their counters during the whole of yesterday were piled up with the packages prepared for their various customers. One gentleman well known on the Change ordered no less than forty boxes of a particular preparation for distribution amongst his servants and friends. The medical men of moderate practice are on the look out for the appointments to the various district boards, which are expected to be tolerably lucrative.[5]

There were other reasons besides jobbery which made the radicals suspect deception in 1832. One member of the Manchester Political Union greeted cholera as 'a mere alarm of the anti-reformers', and *Carpenter's Political Magazine,* in a considered judgement made after the epidemic, acknowledged that cholera was real, but considered a 'hue and cry' had been got up to divert attention from the Reform Bill agitation and the 'misery and wretchedness that everywhere prevail amongst the industrious classes of society'. Many shared the suspicion that cholera was an anti-reform measure.[6] When the third Reform Bill was introduced to a House of Commons reflecting on the rejection of the second Bill by the Lords, and on the riots in Derby, Nottingham and Bristol, one Lambeth doctor reported that: 'A great number of people considered the Sunderland affair as a government hoax got up for the purpose of producing a counter revolutionary excitement...'[7]

Some conservative supporters of aristocratic government did welcome cholera as a diversion from reform. Southey, despairing of the politicians, believed 'the cholera if it comes, which God in his mercy forbid, will be a more effectual ally in aid of the Constitution', and the *British Critic,* an orthodox defender of church and king, preferred 'pestilence, rather than the horrors of revolution and anarchy'.[8] As the government issued its proclamations and regulations in late 1831, the *New Monthly Magazine* raised its elegant and informed drawing room eyebrows and agreed with the radicals:

Truly the proclamation of the Board of Health is something of this character; we do not see what advantage is to attend it, unless it be to frighten people out of their wits, and thus set up cholera as the rival to reform. What if the cholera should be found the only force capable of dissolving the Birmingham Political Union?[9]

If the governing classes ever did think of using cholera as a diversion from reform, their efforts were a singular failure. As the Tory back-room boy, John Wilson Croker, wrote in February, 'Revolution progresses and so does cholera': the radicals prescribed their 'cure' with glee, namely Reform.[10] Thomas Hood included his 'Ode to Malthus' in the *Comic Annual* for the 1832 Christmas gift season and anticipated the welcome which that gentleman would have given to cholera. Such irony was not funny for those who suspected the medical profession and believed that the census taken in the summer of 1831 had been a government enquiry into surplus population. Doherty described the 'amusing logic' of the people in Manchester, 'accustomed to look with distrust on the powers that be...' He approved of the tone though not the conclusions of a logic which had all the flavour of street gossip well informed with the political radicalism stirred up by the Reform Bill agitation. Why have we had no cholera before? the people asked. Why does it come just after the census? Why do the rich show anxiety for the welfare of those they have neglected for so long? It was impossible for a tropical disease to survive so long in the British climate.

> The people, they assert, have been numbered and classified for the purpose of selecting the most populous districts wherein this new disorder might be introduced with the greatest success. The poor are made the victims of it, they contend, for no other reason than that they are found to be too troublesome to their richer neighbours. The parliament have passed acts empowering the local authorities to erect hospitals in the infected districts, to which hospitals all patients are obliged to be removed; and these measures are pronounced to be nothing more than barefaced jobs in the first instance, and a means of removing the poor sick from the sight of their friends so that they may more conveniently be butchered and anatomised by the doctors whose gratuitous services are adduced in confirmation of the accuracy of this view.[11]

The reasoning might be confused, but Malthus, whose views had been accepted by middle-class poor law reformers in the 1820s, was part of the demonology of radical discourse, and was associated with inhumane policies towards the poor which might even include extermination plans for the surplus population.

This reasoning was derived from the sophisticated thinking of working-class radicalism. For others, the response was more primitive but displayed equal contempt for official warnings. In the Newcastle area cholera became the subject of ridicule and people continued their hard drinking. From Glass-Houses, centre of the Tyne glass industry a mile or so below Newcastle Bridge, scenes of excessive drinking were reported in the week before Christmas. When reproved by the local ministers, the people replied, 'We are drinking to keep the cholera away.'[12]

This evidence of lower-class reaction came from the period just before or just after the onset of the epidemic. Whilst it might seem easy to call 'humbug' when told that cholera was coming, it must have been harder to do so when cholera was in the next street or the next room. Yet at the end of July when over a hundred cases had been reported in Manchester, 'the word cholera could not be seriously mentioned in some companies without a man's running the risk of being called a credulous fool or a terrified dupe.'[13] The *Reformer's Gazette* in Glasgow continued to match each day's casualty list with the claim that the cases were 'got up'. Only the huge slaughter of August silenced the *Gazette,* as it silenced most other indicators of working-class feeling on cholera. The radicals again gave clues as to why this attitude persisted. Lovett commented, 'most of the members of our Union had seen enough in Spitalfields and other districts to see that the dreadful disease was caused by want and wretchedness.'[14] In Glasgow, the *Gazette* was even more specific. The cholera deaths of February were a small portion of those —

> who have during the same period died in England from the numerous old and well known evils to which mortal man is obnoxious. The great flood gates of humanity are ever open. Some are hurried through by one disease, some by another. Measles, Scarlett Fever, Typhus, Consumption slay every one its thousands as well as Cholera.[15]

By March, the paper reported over 5,000 recent cases of typhus. The reasons for the lack of a specific lower-class response may be dimly perceived behind these comments. Poverty, sickness and death, and the pain and grief which they brought, were already familiar features of life for the poor and the labouring classes, and cholera was neither more nor less than one more nasty addition to the perils of life in the poorer areas of Britain's towns and cities. When the medical, clerical and other middle-class observers on whom the historian must rely for information reported the 'despondency' and 'fear' on the faces of the population under attack, they perhaps forgot that such fatalism and fear were a

Class, Power and Cholera   101

part of such people's ordinary lives.

(ii) People, Doctors and Boards of Health

What distinguished cholera from the other perils of life was not the danger of the disease itself, but the extraordinary and disturbing way in which the middle and ruling classes were behaving with their rules and regulations, Boards of Health, hospitals and subscriptions. The administrative perspectives of the early chapters described an ill-informed and ill-co-ordinated public health campaign which acted with fragmentary skills and hastily gathered resources and failed in its humanitarian aims — a well-intentioned failure. From the prespective of the working classes these actions looked very different. They provoked a fearful, angry and often violent reaction. This reaction had two sources in working-class experience, their recent unstable relationship with the medical profession, and a set of deeply held feelings which were affronted by insensitive regulations.

The source of the trouble was the medical profession's demand for fresh bodies for dissection. This demand had grown since John Hunter's work in the 1780s. By the 1800s, anatomy and dissection had become a recognised part of a good medical education. The only legal source of 'subjects' was the execution of felons. The rest were supplied by raids on fresh graves made by semi-criminal elements who then sold to the medical schools. This was an open threat to the working-class right to a decent burial. Whatever indignities the poor and working classes suffered in their lives, the one they feared most was the pauper's funeral. If they could, they subscribed to a Friendly Society so their relatives would have money to pay for the funeral and they would have friends to follow the coffin. The satisfaction gained from the decent burial of the dead was threatened by the body-snatchers, as perhaps also were primitive beliefs which associated the resurrection of the dead with the actual body in the ground. Body-snatchers and doctors became a target of popular anger. In 1801, a London mob wrecked a public house used by the resurrection men. In 1803, 1813-14 and 1823, troops had to be called in to protect the Glasgow medical profession and in 1831 the Anatomy Theatre at Aberdeen was pulled down after the discovery of parts of a body nearby. Meanwhile the price of a 'subject' had risen from 4 guineas in 1812 to 10 in 1828. The Burke and Hare murders in Edinburgh and the conviction of a Lancashire anatomy teacher for receiving a body taken from a fresh grave brought public disquiet to a new pitch and by definition made all teaching of anatomy illegal.[16]

The agitation and the petitions which this situation produced faced the government with a serious dilemma. If they asserted their traditional role and defended popular rights, then they brought serious medical education to a halt. If they continued with the existing compromise of public disapproval and private acquiescence over body-snatching, then popular violence would increase. Many members of the ruling classes were prepared to defend popular rights without reservation. 'Every man in this country', said the Earl of Harewood, 'has a right to a Christian burial when dead.' He co-operated with men like Michael Thomas Sadler, evangelical MP and protagonist of factory reform. All attempts to reach a compromise were delayed. Those who supported an Act which would bring a regulated supply of bodies to the medical schools claimed that they, too, were acting in the interests of the poor. The inexperienced newly qualified surgeon, they pointed out, frequently began his career treating the poor, usually as the Poor Law surgeon. Thus it was in the interest of the poor that he should be properly trained.[17] The Philosophical Radicals gave wholehearted support to an Anatomy Bill. Science-based knowledge and education was of more value to them than traditional values, but with their keen sense of social structure they saw that popular resentment was based on class discrimination. As the wealthier families began to guard their graves with man-traps, iron cages and patrols in their graveyards, the greater vulnerability of the poor became obvious. It was not surprising that the poor were angry at the appearance of their relatives in the dissecting room —

> They often feel deeply and in the bitterness of wounded spirit, execrate the hardness of their lot; they imagine, it must be owned with some colour of reason, that they live only for the rich; this detestable practice [body snatching] leads them to suppose that they must still serve their masters even after death has set them free from toil, and that when the early dawn can no longer rouse them from their pallet of straw to work, they must be dragged from what should be their last bed, to show in common with the murderer, how the knife of the surgeon may best avoid the rich man's artery, and least afflict the rich man's nerve.[18]

The Anatomy Act became law in 1832. It made available to the medical schools, the bodies of those who had died in work-houses, prisons and hospitals, unless these bodies were claimed by friends or relatives and unless the individual had made specific objection before his death. Parliament compromised between popular feeling and professional need by drawing a distinction between those with friends and those with no friends. Although the Act did a great deal to cool the conflict between people and doctors, the events of the previous thirty years left a deep popular distrust of the profession.

In light of their recent experience and expectations of the medical profession and their deep feelings over burial customs, the working classes could only be alarmed by the regulations which the Privy Council prepared for isolation in hospitals and the burial of cholera victims. The contagionist victory at the Board of Health meant a policy of separating the sick from the healthy.

The 13 December regulations directed that as 'space, cleanliness and pure air' were the best aids to recovery, a patient should be isolated in a room in his own house with as few people in contact with him as possible, or 'be induced to submit to an immediate removal to such building as may have been provided for the reception of persons whose circumstances will not afford the advantages at home of space, air and separation from the healthy'. This from the best motives meant the removal of poor and labouring-class cholera patients to hospital and the nursing of wealthier ones at home.

Prejudice against cholera hospitals was a major problem in all parts of the country. No one wanted the hospital in their area of town. No one wanted to go into hospital. The hospital ship H.M.S. *Dover* was sent to Limehouse Reach but found that patients only came in a state verging on collapse. In Edinburgh, the Board of Health agreed that hospital treatment was the best for all concerned, but that it could not be enforced as this would encourage people to conceal cases.[19] In Manchester, Gaulter found that the poor never overcame their fear of hospital and only entered one to prevent infection spreading to the rest of the family, or because of pressure from neighbours:

> ...the scene which followed the announcement of the van was often most distressing: while the neighbours insisted on removal, the relations would refuse to allow it, and support their refusal by a denial of the nature of the disease, the poor victim himself suffering during the noisy conflict and aggravation of that despair, which is one of the most constant and most fatal features of the disease.[20]

Both Doherty and Cobbett knew that the poor man's fear of hospital was based on the belief that he would be murdered and dissected by the doctors. In the early days of the epidemic the action of many doctors only strengthened this fear. Anxious to increase their knowledge of the new disease they carried out rapid autopsies of the dead with scant

regard for the wishes or feelings of relatives. The early correspondence
of the Central Board was full of post-mortem reports, until the Board
advised doctors to proceed with more caution to avoid discontent.[21]
The hospitals themselves were unsuitable, inefficient and uninviting
buildings. Some were temporary buildings, others damp and chill,
warehouses, schoolrooms, tents, and one was in a steam laundry in the Isle
of Dogs. Although the administrators and medical men believed that
hospital treatment was better than leaving a patient in the crowded and
filthy rooms in which many of them lived, they recognised that the
policy did more harm than good because most patients only came in
the collapse stage of the disease, and had to be carried through the chill
streets in a rattling, swaying cholera van:

> the terror inspired by even a brief incarceration in such a place (to
> say nothing of the vibrating motion of the carriage, of the semi-
> nudity in which the carelessness of the assistants often left the
> patient, or of the filthiness of the blankets in which he was wrapped
> defiled by successive occupants) – that terror was found to work as
> might be anticipated a change for the worse....[22]

Even those who operated the hospitals with caution and sensitivity
realised that the system was regarded with anxious resentment as an
attack on the family as the social unit which could and should care for
its members. On 19 July, the Oxford Board of Health was told that a
father had asked to enter the cholera hospital to see if it was 'suitable'
for his child. The request had been referred to the Board which
unfortunately did not record its decision.[23] In Sunderland, Haslewood
and Mordey found: 'The wife of the most wretched pauper thinks she
can make him more comfortable with his ragged blanket than all the
luxuries of a hospital without her.'[24] It is a pity that the nature of the
evidence available means that of these quiet attempts to act upon family
loyalties and affections, few were recorded. Reactions to the cholera
hospitals highlighted attitudes that must have been common to all
hospitals and suggest that their failings, however great or small, were
not only as medical units but also as social units which could gain the
confidence and co-operation of their patients.

The burial regulations were a scientifically-based administrative
attack on the burial and mourning customs of the poor and working
classes:

> Those who died of this disease should be buried as soon as possible,

wrapped in cotton or linen cloth saturated with pitch, or coal tar, and be carried to the grave by the fewest possible number of persons. The funeral service to be performed in the open air.

If possible, the victims were to be buried in detached ground adjoining the cholera hospital. Local Boards enforced these provisions with varying degrees of severity. At Leith the poor were hurried to their graves at dawn. In St Anne's, Middlesex, the early victims were wrapped in blankets dipped in coal tar and buried in a coffin filled with lime. The use of quicklime by several local authorities was seen to 'outrage the feelings of the poor, especially the Irish'. The Parish Clerk of St Stephen's Coleman Lane remembered very tangible reasons for the objections of the poor. The bodies decomposed rapidly and became semi-liquid as they were carried along, '...there was a discharge from the coffin...I cannot describe how that coffin smelt.'[25] Besides, quicklime was another association with the burial of felons. Above all, a working-class funeral needed time. Relatives often kept bodies in their crowded homes for several days while they sought money for undertakers, mourning clothes and funeral teas. Then they would wait until Sunday, so that friends and relatives would be free from work and able to attend. Many, especially the Irish, observed the ritual of a drunken wake around the body. The Central Board of Health insisted that funerals should take place within 24 hours, thus disrupting these traditional burial customs, 'their bit of pride' and adding anger and dismay to grief. In public health terms there were good reasons for doing so. One purpose of laying out the body in the room or house in which the family lived was so that family and friends could pay their last respects to the body itself. The lower down the social scale and the nearer to Scotland and to Ireland, the more likely this was to involve direct physical contact. Janet Lindsay, the 'old woman very much addicted to the use of whiskey' died in the Goosedubbs, early in the Glasgow epidemic. Over 50 people attended her and stayed behind to help dress the body. Physical contact with the dead was a major outlet and expression of grief which had been brought to the poor by causes they could neither understand nor control. As one undertaker recalled in 1842:

> I have seen a child which has died of smallpox, which perhaps has been dead eight or ten days, and the face completely black, and all I could do would not keep the mother from kissing that child.[26]

Such physical contact must have greatly increased the opportunities for a water-borne infection like cholera to spread. The conflict of popular and administrative values was nowhere greater than over the burial of the dead.

Rev. William Leigh of Bilston, who thought out his response to an explosive local epidemic with special care, found that the members of the benefit clubs were no longer following the coffin and reluctantly decided to forbid cholera burials in family graves. His wish to avoid contagion overrode religious and popular pressure; 'I tremble', he wrote, 'for the effect it might produce among the lower classes of my parishioners.'[27] At Exeter, resistance to the burial regulations caused rioting. The crowd resented above all the use of land other than traditional consecrated ground.[28] Resistance was mainly at an individual level. In Oxford, a widow of St Aldates was fined £5 for re-interring the body of her husband after he had died of cholera.[29] There was a squalid little incident in August, in Seven Dials, which showed all the conflict of authority, custom and fear created by the regulations. The relatives refused to allow burial. The magistrate ordered the police to remove the body as a danger to public health. The police refused. The commissioners (presumably a local improvement commission) asked the magistrate for special constables, but the Beadle told him: 'the parish couldn't git a special constable no how; none of the householders wouldn't serve.' In the end, thirty watermen were marched up from Strand Lane and seven of them carried away the body for 5s. each.[30]

In many cases there was a sinister finale to the clinical history of cholera which only increased fears of being buried alive, murdered by doctors, and perhaps worst, of being dissected alive. In early 1832, the London papers reported that a labourer had been buried alive at Haddington. He was given up for dead by the doctors, but five hours later swept the grave clothes from himself. No notice was taken and he was buried in a few fir boards hastily nailed together. The chairman of the Haddington Board of Health denied the report and criticised it as 'of a nature likely to prejudice the minds of the ignorant'. There had been a convulsive action of the head and hip as the body was being prepared for burial. The attendants had kept the body warm and left it for an hour and a half with no result.[31] Convulsions like this gave cholera one of its many names, spasmodic cholera. Readers of the reviews and the medical periodicals already knew what to expect from the reports from Russia and by the summer of 1832 most doctors were familiar with movements like those described by the York doctor, Charles Anderson:

Class, Power and Cholera

> Our attention has frequently been called to these [movements] by the nurses, who were exceedingly alarmed in many instances. They usually commence about a quarter of an hour after death, and increase in violence for upwards of an hour...it is always the most violent in those in whom the cramps have been the most severe, and have died rapidly. The whole leg, from the hip occasionally, moves upwards for at least six or seven inches, at which time all the muscles are in tremulous motion, and the toes in constant action. I think it affects the lower much more than the upper extremities. We have taken particular notice of a slight return of heat a short time before death...'[32]

Other writers described movements of the head, neck and hands like convulsions during galvanism. These movements, like the return of heat to the body at death, all increased suspicion.

There were a host of minor matters in which administrative aims and the feelings of the poor came into conflict. The endless house-to-house visitations, whitewashing, cleansing and destruction of infected clothing and bedding, all appear by the science-based values of the Board of Health as essential and responsible measures to stop the spread of infection. Many pamphlets recorded the gratitude of the poor, and many must have been grateful for help given. The pamphlet-writers were eager to celebrate the work done by local doctors and boards of health and naturally did not record the attitudes expressed by Cobbett.

> I must insist that he [the Lord Mayor of London] send no more messengers (for whose services I dare say I shall have to pay) to inquire into the state of my rooms, kitchen, cellar, dust hole and water courses.[33]

Doherty complained about the plight of a local family afflicted by cholera. All their clothes and furniture were burnt and he appealed for a replacement fund to help them.[34] Some local boards do seem to have made compensation. The Oxford accounts included an item of £17.5s.11d. for 'goods destroyed'. This was distributed to people like Mrs Sidley who appeared before the Board on 5 July to demand compensation for bedding which had been burnt. By the 12th the burning, and the expense and the discontent it led to, had been stopped.[35] As with the early development of welfare legislation at the beginning of the twentieth century, the working classes did not always welcome state action, much of it taken to protect their health and welfare. The action of the state was interpreted in the light of previous experience, mainly with the Poor Law authorities, and in practice state action was an interference with privacy and a disruption of the precarious home life which poverty allowed.[36]

(iii) The Riots

In many places the public health measures of the authorities and the doctors met violent and extensive popular resistance. There was a wave of rioting in March–April 1832 as the epidemic began to spread, a serious riot in Manchester in late summer and a host of minor incidents in which doctors and Boards of Health were threatened.

In late March 1832, Parliament heard with concern that a mob of Irish people had prevented the parish authorities from burying the body of a woman and child who had died in the Grosvenor Square area of London. The husband, a man called Sanderland, claimed that his wife had been in labour, and the authorities had called it cholera so they might remove the body rapidly. Sanderland paid for his defiance, for within a few days both he and his son were dead from cholera. Neighbours and friends kept the authorities out and a huge concourse of people escorted the bodies to Bayswater Cemetery.[37] The funeral was followed by a mob attack on the cholera hospital of St George's in the East, which was only stopped by the quick thinking of the surgeon in charge. He pulled the mob leader forcibly inside, made him talk to the patients and then tell the crowd outside what he had seen. The crowd dispersed on hearing that the patients were well treated.[38] Less fortunate was the old man being carried by a surgeon and his assistant to the Mary-le-bone hospital. He was seized by a crowd said to number 6,000 and carried naked through the night back to his own house 'saved from being "burked"'. The medical men tried to recover their patient, but the accommodation chair was taken from them and they were pelted with the pieces. The police restored order, albeit at the cost of injury to one constable of D Division, who was felled with a warming pan.

Opposition was more violent and widespread in Scotland than in England. The local boards met the same threats, insults and half-bricks as James Arthur and his men had done in the winter. When cholera appeared in the Edinburgh suburban village of the Water of Leith, the Edinburgh Board, worried by the consequences of people ignoring their instructions, issued new notices in the Press and set up a quarantine hospital in Fountainbridge, much to local alarm and resentment. The cholera van was attacked as it returned to Fountainbridge from carrying a sick man to the cholera hospital at Castlehill. The van was wrecked and tipped in the canal and the windows of the two hospitals broken. Although the crowd was described as 'the lowest rabble by which the streets are infested', the leader who seized the van was a baker, and the areas involved were those inhabited by journeymen and tradesmen, not the Canongate area which held the poorest population of Edinburgh.[39] The following Saturday, Main Street in Gorbals was filled with a crowd of 1,500 to 2,000 people, 'composed of Irish labourers, blackguard boys and ill-tongued women', who stopped the surgeon reaching Elizabeth Fulton, 'an old dissipated female', well known in the Bridewell. She was suffering from cholera. Mr Stewart took shelter with a shopkeeper who acted bravely in view of the damage this might do to his local reputation. The mob pelted the medical men with mud and stones, shouting 'medical murderer', 'cholera humbug' and 'Burkers' The police eventually made a way for the surgeon but the woman had died, not before a rumour had spread through the crowd that when the surgeon was forcing drugs down her throat, a drop fell on a cloth and burnt right through.[40]

The worst rioting took place a week later in Paisley. Two small shovels and a hook on the end of a piece of cord were found by two boys playing under a bridge on the way to the cholera burial ground on Paisley Moss. These tools of the body-snatching trade were displayed in the town and by afternoon the coffins at the burial ground were being opened and crowds running across the fields to see the results. Six out of seven coffins were found empty and the crowd returned to town, bearing an empty coffin on their shoulders and threatening vengeance on the doctors. The magistrates offered a £50 reward for the body-snatchers but this failed to stop the riot. The police were swept aside and the crowd went systematically from street to street smashing the windows and shops of all the doctors in the town, with the exception of a Dr Stewart, who was cheered in the mistaken belief that he had denied the existence of cholera. The gates of the cholera hospital in School Wynd were forced, and the cholera van carried away and broken up. The only death in the cholera rioting occurred here when a patient was struck on the head by a stone. For this attack two chimney sweeps were arrested. The crowd did not disperse until late afternoon when a troop of the 4th Dragoons arrived from Glasgow. The troops were not used directly, but provided a show of force to back the arguments of police and bailies. Although the lower classes of Paisley had taken advantage of their distance from the military to take complete control of the town, the damage they did, apart from a few stray missiles which hit the Trades Library, was limited to the doctors who were the specific target of their anger.[41] The surgeons retaliated by resigning *en masse* from the local Board of Health, thus cutting off free medical treatment. One of the crowd leaders who had dug up some of the coffins died of cholera a few days later, cursing his surgeon and denying he had the disease. 'To complete the drama, the family buried him themselves, and then commenced drinking freely — to the alarm of the whole neighbourhood, and the certain danger of the whole town.'[42] The family had done everything which brute strength and their narrow experience could do to defend themselves and those like them against the unjustifiable actions of the doctors. Then in the moment of victory they had been defeated totally and without recourse by a microorganism of which neither they nor their persecutors knew.

After that, the authorities were more careful but in September they failed to prevent a riot in Manchester. Between five and six o'clock in the evening of 2 September, the streets in New Cross and St George's Road were filled with a crowd of several thousand, carrying a coffin containing the headless body of a four-year-old boy. The boy had lost both his parents and was being cared for by his grandfather, John Hase. The old man had been told that the boy was recovering from cholera on the Friday. Next day he was refused admission to Swan Street Hospital. On application to the Board of Health, he was told his grandson was dead. He went with friends and raised the coffin and found that the boy's head had been removed and replaced with a brick, thus confirming his suspicion that the boy had been a victim of the anatomists. The crowd brought the coffin through the main streets of Manchester. In Oldham Street, they met Robert Sharpe, surgeon, who was compelled to dismount from his gig and inspect the body. 'The cries of execration against the doctors were very general, and an almost unanimous shout, "To the hospital, pull it to the ground", took place.' When the crowd arrived at Swan Street, they broke the windows, pulled down the yard wall and forced the gates. The patients were liberated, and many taken back to their homes by the invaders. Some walked out. Others collapsed and died. Inside the hospital, beds, furniture and bedding were smashed and seized. One of the spring vehicles for carrying patients to the hospital was broken into fragments. The other was saved by the arrival of police armed with cutlasses. This so angered the crowd that they attacked the police lock-up close to the hospital. Messengers were then sent to Hulme Barracks and Lord Brudenell arrived with four troops of the 15th Hussars. They arrested the ringleaders and nine men were escorted to the New Bailey. With this force at their backs, the magistrates were able to disperse the crowd by reading the Riot Act.[43] The crowd was 'principally of the lower classes' and most of those arrested were Irish. This was to be expected because of the location of the riot. Between Swan Street and the River Irk was 'Irish Town', an area heavily marked with cholera cases on Gaulter's map, an area of crowded cottages and tenement housing inhabited by hand loom weavers and workers in the noxious trades (dye-works, gas-works, tanneries, bone manufactories, size manufactories and tripe houses) which added to the unhealthiness of the area. This was not the worst area of Manchester. The streets west of Deansgate, the quarter inhabited by 'prostitutes and thieves', was the worst, but Irish Town held the lowest strata of the wage-earning population.[44] The people still had the self-respect of earning an honest living (just) in conditions of appalling insecurity, and thus the self-respect to defend their rights against the authorities. Besides, they were on the opposite side of Manchester to Hulme Barracks, a minor but important factor when the military was the only effective method of crowd control.

The discovery of the mutilated body of the boy had been the spark which started the riot, but this was not the whole story. Doherty's *Poor Man's Advocate* had reported crowds 'found nightly grumbling around the cholera hospital in Swan Street', long before the riot.[45] Tension had mounted since March. As Mrs Perry wept over the grave of her recently dead husband, it had been whispered to her that the body was no longer there but had been 'resurrected' by a medical man, the brother of Mr Gilpin, a Stockport parson. Popular memory went back to the mangled body of the Irishman which had recently been found in the Dispensary. Gilpin denied all knowledge and Doherty found himself in Lancaster Jail for libel, without being allowed by the court to bring any defence. This case kept one of the major radical papers of Manchester discussing the threat of the medical profession to the bodies of the poor and the possibility that cholera could be an excuse for further indignities. In this atmosphere, the discovery of the headless body was enough to spark off the riot.

The riots followed a familiar pattern. They all occurred in areas with active medical schools, where the population had been angered by body-snatching. Many of the crowds were Irish-dominated, for their burial customs suffered most disruption from the regulations. Although large crowds dominated important streets for several hours at a time, the violence was limited and controlled, a fact which the radicals threw in the faces of the 'liberal' newspapers which referred to the 'ignorant rabble'.[46] Violence was directed at the specific targets of their anger.

Even then property was only deliberately smashed when the hospitals and doctors' houses were attacked. Even the surgeon caught in the Manchester crowd was only harassed.

The ruling class, through the Central Board of Health acting as a committee of the Privy Council, responded to the violence and anger of the poor and working classes in the traditional manner, by taking action to cool the potential conflict and control the actions of their own agents and middlemen, in this case the medical profession, which threatened to disrupt social stability. European experience had warned the Privy Council that anti-cholera measures could cause popular violence. The activities of Russell and Barry in Moscow had been cut short by mob action which had been especially directed at foreign doctors. The Russian 'lower classes' believed that no such disease as cholera existed, but that the epidemic was produced by poison administered by the doctors in order to reduce a population which had become too numerous to be easily governed. This plan, the people claimed, had been successfully used by the British in India and was being copied by the Russians. In Moscow, hospitals were sacked, patients released and several doctors murdered. When cholera reached Hungary the rumour spread that wells were being poisoned. This was probably a result of the sacks of chlorate of lime which were tipped into water supplies in a desperate attempt to purify them. In several areas armed bands of peasants went from village to village murdering any physicians and nobles they could find.[47]

The Central Board of Health had started the summer of 1831 with a strong policy of isolating the sick and their contacts in hospitals, but on considering European events and British tradition, they rejected coercion for internal quarantine, for hospitals and even for cleansing. When challenged on their weakness, Poulett-Thompson told the Commons that coercion would arouse too much opposition: 'He would put it to any gentleman, whether he thought that considering the habits of the British people they would submit to such a system for one week?'[48] The Central Board made considerable concessions on hospitals and quarantine but were less moved by the opposition to the burial regulations. In July 1832 they confirmed the 24 hours maximum time allowed for the burial of cholera victims. The response may have been weaker because popular violence was less aroused by this issue. During the epidemic, the Central Board frequently acted to ensure that local boards were equally restrained. In Leeds, where one physician had already been attacked in an isolated incident, the Board was warned, 'the general prejudice existing on the part of the lower classes to be removed to the cholera hospitals [is such] that no compulsory measures should be used...'.[49] Special care was taken with Sunderland. The doctors were naturally anxious to learn more about the new disease, but their lack of caution was counter-productive. The presence of many foreigners only added to local suspicions and many visitors noted the poor relations between local people and doctors. When the Central Board learned of this situation through the reports of Dr Daun, they sent a sharp order through him that all dissections were to stop unless the doctors had the relative's permission. This order was made publicly known.[50] Others realised the need to compromise with popular prejudice without the prompting of London. In Oxford, the Board rejected the idea of using coercion to get people into hospital and even Warburton, MP and passionate supporter of the medical profession and the Anatomy Act, had objected when the body of an early London cholera victim was put on public display to the 'gratification of idle curiosity'.[51]

The authorities reacted to violence and the possibility of violence in a traditional manner. The pattern of interaction was known and expected by both sides; an infringement of a mutually recognised popular right by a middleman − threats of violence from the crowd − a ruling-class response to restore popular rights without compromising their own authority. This pattern was familiar in the eighteenth century when the 'law-giving mob' had used force of numbers to bring down grain prices in years of poor harvest. Violence was normally limited and controlled and in some cases riot leaders saw that the grain dealers were paid at a 'fair' price fixed by the crowd. These riots were violent and dangerous but very different in their morality from the burning and looting of twentieth-century city riots or the senseless destruction of the Bristol riots in 1831. The name of the crowd which terrorised farmers in the Thames Valley in 1766, 'the Regulators', expressed the social purposes of these crowds and the government recognised this purpose in their response. Troops were sent to the area affected by riots but rarely clashed with crowds. Their presence was often accompanied by action to persuade middlemen to release grain supplies at 'fair' prices. This limited violence derived, not so much from the organisation of the crowd, but from common notions of fairness in their relationships with grain dealers, employers and their rulers. By the end of the century, pressure on food supplies and the tension between aristocratic government and radical political demands meant that the temperate use of violence as an element in class relationships became harder to maintain. The events in Swan Street and Paisley showed that the law-giving mob could still operate in 1832.[52]

The limited extent of the cholera riots and the manner in which they were controlled were indicators of the inherent stability of British society. The class relationships revealed by cholera showed the expectations each class had of the other's likely response in given situations. The accepted legitimacy of certain responses in those situations meant that the conflict arising out of the impact of cholera could be resolved without the full involvement of the main force resources which both sides in the conflict had at their disposal. There was none of the uncontrolled and extended violence of Moscow, Hungary or Paris. Where troops were used, they never clashed with the crowd but merely provided a visible presence to back the magistrates reading the Riot Act. British society had developed such confrontations to a dangerous ritual of riot − military presence − magistrates or bailies taking action − dispersal of crowd. It was a ritual in which the real forces of crowd violence and military strength were matched against each other without being brought into contact. The riots at Manchester, Paisley, Glasgow, Edinburgh and in London which have been examined were themselves abnormalities in this relationship between rulers and ruled. More typical were the examples of Sunderland, Leeds and Oxford. Indeed the debate within the Central Board of Health during summer 1831, when their anti-cholera plans were laid, was guided by principles of avoiding conflict, and respecting popular rights, whilst maintaining social stability and their own authority. At this level the main force elements of military and crowd were never visible but nevertheless had a real part to play in the decisions made. The stability with which this ritualised and latent main force confrontation worked in the cholera epidemic was more remarkable as it took place at the end of the Reform Bill agitation of 1831-2 in which this stable main force relationship had broken down, troops had clashed with crowds, the authority of the ruling class was compromised, to be painfully reassembled in the political manoeuvrings of the following decades. The ability and willingness of the government to compromise with popular prejudice during the epidemic was one reason for the weakness of government authority in countering the epidemic and improving public health. The weakness was not only caused by merchant pressure groups anxious for their cargoes, but also by a fear of popular violence around burial grounds and hospitals.

(iv) Communications Problems

The confusion and suspicion of the lower classes was increased by two minor communication difficulties faced by the authorities. The nineteenth century was the high point of the era of government by wall poster in Britain. What had begun as an occasional notice pinned to the church door by parish and county authorities had, by 1830, with the advent of cheap printing, developed into a flood of instructions, regulations, explanations, advertisements and political, philanthropic and personal pleas, in a thousand causes, petty and important. In the 1970s, all that is left of a once vital media of communication are the anonymous surrogates of the advertising world and the pale survival which confronts us at parliamentary and local elections. Only the graffiti of the vandals shows that a media killed by radio and television is still alive as a folk art. During the cholera epidemics the handbills and posters showered a wide range of information, regulation and warning on an anxious population. The Edinburgh Board of Health was very conscious of the function of the handbill.

> We have besides circulated very extensively among the lower orders, various handbills, informing them of the arrangements of the Board for their welfare and instructing them how to proceed, so as to procure immediate relief for their sick friends.[53]

These posters made numerous attempts to change and direct the behaviour of the poor and back up the voluntary public health policy. People affected by cholera were asked to seek early treatment and were given lists of stations at which help could be found. They were encouraged to come into hospitals fitted up at great expense, staffed by experienced people, and promised that 'under the blessings of Providence' many thousands of lives would be saved. Other handbills aroused neighbourhood fears of infection and noted that hospitals eliminated the danger to friends and neighbours. Edinburgh people were asked not to visit infected places along the Forth and warned of the dangers they were exposed to 'by indulging to excess in the use of strong liquors, especially ardent spirits'. They were regaled with the story of the three Warsaw butchers who drank themselves insensible in a tavern and were dead within four hours of being carried home, as well as numerous other salutary tales from Europe. G.H. Bell sent a collection of these handbills to his friend Dr Buckland for the use of the Oxford Board of Health. Oxford produced its own pleas for entry to hospital, and sobriety at St Giles' Fair as well as a detailed list of recommended medicines, cleansing measures and information about supplies of lime.[54] The early debate over the presence and nature of cholera in Sunderland was conducted by handbill as well as by press report and letter. The same debate took place on the hoardings of Newcastle in the following month, appeals, denials and derision.[55]

Despite the weight of information and entreaty directed at the lower classes, their response was minimal. Hospitals were empty, relatives in infected areas were visited, and the taverns, markets and fairs were, with few exceptions, as busy and lacking in sobriety as usual. Cobbet greeted this mass of advice with derision and many other readers must have done likewise. Gaulter criticised the bills for increasing anxiety during the epidemic with little real purpose:

> Without any adequate counterbalance of benefit, these systems committed the capital offence of setting and keeping at work, through a whole community, that agitation and fear which, as we have seen, rendered the human frame most capable of being acted upon by the cause of cholera. The perpetual appearance of fresh placards headed by this dreadful word – (as well as funerals and cholera vans) – all this ostentation of pestilence was most pernicious.[56]

The response to this information and instruction was patchy and often hostile, sometimes resulting in increasing fear and suspicion. Yet if the partial knowledge of cholera which the authorities possessed in 1832 was to be of any value to those most at risk, it had to come to them via the media of the wall poster. The very nature of this media made its partial success inevitable. Though the working classes of Britain were by no means illiterate, around 30 per cent of them were unable to read or write,[57] and those in the poorest sections of the working class, the Irish, the inhabitants of crowded housing, or members of the declining trades were most likely to be found in that 30 per cent. Thus the handbill, the literary medium, was a realistic means of communication between the authorities and the bulk of the working population, but those sections of Britain's population most at risk in the cholera epidemic were least likely to be able to read the instructions of the Board, or perhaps worse, received partial, alarmist impressions from the second-hand reports they gained from friends and neighbours and their own ability to puzzle out a few words.

Matters were made worse by the very obvious source of the cholera posters. The evaluation of any communication is affected not only by the receiver's technical mastery of the media but by his expectation and trust of the sender. The senders were the local boards of health.

The composition of these boards would not inspire the confidence of the poor. In Edinburgh 14 out of 27 members were medical men, and another three were managers of the Royal Infirmary, not a majority designed to secure popular trust in the city of Burke and Hare.[58] In the Leeds Board, politics added to popular mistrust. Seventeen of the 56 members were from the closed Corporation, Tory, Anglican and target of popular radical leaders campaigning for parliamentary reform.[59] In addition there were 17 doctors, physicians and surgeons, several from the Poor Law service. Seven of the remainder were either church wardens or trustees of the workhouse, men closely associated with the administration of the workhouse. Others, like Baines and Cawood, had recently been heavily involved in workhouse politics. Their knowledge of administration and resources was just what the cholera board wanted, but they associated the local boards with the Poor Law, which was an institution which aroused special mistrust among the poor and working classes. It represented a special threat to their personal freedom. The workhouse office was the daily scene of perpetual and degrading disputes over doles and conditions of residence in the workhouse. When individuals arrived at cholera hospitals and stations seeking help, many details would remind them of the Poor Law. In Oxford, when the Board looked for menus for the cholera hospital, they immediately applied to the workhouse and adopted their diet sheets. The workhouse was the only experience which local leadership had in institutional feeding and hence the easiest place for them to turn for advice. The rates were raised by the same means as the poor rates; even Mr Welton, the workhouse beadle, turned up, to keep order at funerals.[60]

(v) The Middle Classes

The working-class response was basically one of mistrust for their rulers. Middle-class response was more complex. Fear, panic and apathy have been ascribed to them, whilst they claimed they acted with all social responsibility.

Although fear of the working class as a source of disease was a developing aspect of class relationships in 1832, in practice this fear was visited during the cholera epidemic on a particular section of the working class. Itinerant labourers, tramps, hawkers and vagrants were a conspicuous and distasteful part of the labouring classes, many of them begging on doorsteps and street corners or tramping along the high road. They were seen for what indeed they must have been, an ideal way of transmitting disease from one centre to another. Several of the first cases were vagrants and travellers. Many places took action to exclude vagrants by setting watches on the road. In Newcastle the police drove them out. In Oxford the Mendicity societies were used. Cheltenham excluded over 2,000 vagrants. They were escorted around the outskirts, given relief and sent on their way. Cheltenham escaped, thus safeguarding its reputation as a resort — one of the few English examples of successful internal quarantine. The constables of Liberton, outside Edinburgh, were instructed 'to hinder as much as possible the wandering of beggars throughout the parish'. The Scottish authorities were very active in moving vagrants from the urban centres and this may have encouraged the spread of cholera to villages which was much greater than south of the border.[61] One popular guide on cholera protection advised its readers — 'avoid beggars, vagabonds, old clothes men, smugglers and all liable to bring infection. Indeed, every village ought to be cleared of them'.[62] In several places the Board of Health issued handbills asking householders not to give relief to any beggars but send them to the vagrant office or the local soup kitchen. The movement of vagrants and itinerant labourers was the only aspect of internal communication which was seriously attacked during the epidemic. The stage-coaches, the carriers' carts, the canals and most coastal shipping moved freely. The tramp and the beggar were driven away because they were a visible source of infection. In many ways this campaign was illogical for it helped spread disease. More relevant was a request made to the Poor Law Unions to stop the removal of paupers from one parish to another.[63]

Other links in the chain of human contact which spread cholera were markets, fairs and traditional festivals. Although these were viewed with suspicion, they were generally allowed to continue unhindered. In Scotland, Old Handsel Monday hastened the spread of cholera along the Forth. It was part of the traditional New Year celebration. Relatives visited each other, drank whisky and as the *Cholera Gazette* reported:

> . . .last Monday, being the first Monday of the year, old style, or, as it is called, "Old Handsel Monday" was a day of great festivity and rejoicing among the lower orders of society in this part of the country; and many of the unfortunate cases which have occurred yesterday and today, may, I fear, in a great measure be attributed to intoxication, and exposure to the atmospherical air while in that state.[64]

Whit Monday, 28 May, which was flitting day in Glasgow, had a similar effect. Furniture and bundles of clothes were carted across the poorer areas of the City, and cholera spread to previously uninfected districts. The upsurge in cases 14 days after was attributed to the unpacking of clothes which had carried infection with them.[65] In the Black Country the explosive outbreaks at Tipton and Bilston came just after the local wakes weeks.[66] In Oxford, the local Board considered stopping St Giles' Fair but realised that such a prohibition could never be enforced and had to be satisfied with notices about the consequences of drink. These fairs and festivals were associated with crime, drink, licentiousness and disorder and were thus a natural object of 'respectable' opprobrium even before cholera came. These fairs and festivals did play a minor part in the spread of cholera, but most of the infection was carried by the day-to-day contact of a commercial and industrial economy, the labourers and vagrants moving from one urban centre to another in search of work. The weavers of Kirkintilloch taking their work to the merchants of Glasgow, the fishermen of the north-east coast selling their wares in nearby towns, weekly markets, carriers' carts, colliers along the coast, hawkers and visitors of all kinds. Cholera was always worst where poor drainage and this type of contact went together. Birmingham escaped because it was well drained, Cheltenham because the local economy allowed the links to be cut. The ports like Newcastle, Liverpool and Glasgow were most vulnerable.

In 1832, the middle class organised and acted as a class at local and provincial level but rarely operated on a national basis except as allies of an aristocratic faction. At local level their most characteristic response was to raise and distribute a voluntary subscription for the relief of the poor during the epidemic. In Leeds, nearly £5,000 was raised, in Oxford just over £800. In practical terms the work of the local boards, dominated by medical and Poor Law men, was most important, but the voluntary funds were more significant as an expression of class feeling. In many cases, the funds were needed to overcome the cumbersome delays of an outdated structure of local government. They were a result of the middle-class adoption of the paternalistic values of the eighteenth-century aristocracy as they consolidated their urban power. Their privilege and authority were legitimised, at least in their own eyes, by their ability to defend the 'rights', as they saw them, and protect the living standards of poorer classes. An ideal of duty and responsibility guided the actions of many individuals during the epidemic. Robert Southey roused himself to take part in the Keswick Board of Health. Despite pleas and invitations from friends to stay with them in the safety of the Yorkshire coastal resort of Scarborough, James Montgomery stopped in Sheffield to act on the local Board of Health.[67] It also followed from the poverty theory of cholera which became increasingly prominent in official and medical advice that bread, soup, blankets and other doles would reduce the spread of infection and protect the rest of the community.

When Edward Baines appealed for funds in Leeds, he admitted that subscribers would have a double motive of duty and interest. Others agreed with him:

> To the opulent and easy classes of the community we should therefore appeal, if it were only for their own safety, not to mention the nobler motive of charity; we should entreat them to think often of the poor who everywhere surround us, and who must be everywhere, ill-clad, ill-fed, ill-housed, and exposed to that constant depression of mind, which, more than any other circumstance, invites and encourages the malady. Soups may be made for them at little cost; warm clothing especially flannels, may be provided for them in abundance by very small subscriptions; coals and wood and lime for whitewashing their apartments might through the same means be supplied to them, at least during the approaching winter, and until all danger of cholera shall have passed away.[68]

Others were not so kind about middle-class motives for these subscriptions:

> The wretch who might have died in squalid want
> Unseen, unmourned by our hard hearted blindness
> Wringing from fear what pity would not grant
> Becomes the sudden object of kindness
> Now that his betters he may implicate
> And spread infection to the rich and great
>
> O thou reforming cholera! thou'rt sent
> Not as a scourge alone but as a teacher[69]

It was not true as this implied that relief funds were new or were restricted to cholera. In Leeds, and most other towns, they had been raised during every trade depression since the beginning of the century. They were a well-tried method of alleviating the discontent of poverty. Such memories did not curb the scorn of people like Cobbett:

> It is curious to see how this great vessel is rocking to and fro, and

how at every lurch, the poor and oppressed part of the people *gain something!* The RICH are now raising money, nay, the law is about to make them pay money, to supply the means of giving proper food, raiment, bedding, medicines and fuel, to the *POOR!*...
Why was not this done *before?* Because before *the rich were in no danger* from contagion existing amongst the poor![70]

Hetherington greeted the rising subscriptions of November with contempt and hoped that the plague would last long enough for the poor to be fed throughout the winter. By February he complained that the increasing acceptance of non-contagionist views was reducing the level of subscriptions.[71] Doherty dismissed some of the subscriptions in the Manchester areas as a re-re-distribution of income. For example, £20 had come from the Salford fustian manufacturer, Lawrence Rostron. Now Rostron Brothers had just reduced their wages from ten to seven shillings a piece, which with a labour force of 100, meant that the liberal subscription represented a week's savings on the wages cut:

> The process seems to be, to deprive the poor wretches of wages, that Mr. Rostron may gain the credit of being liberal and benevolent in giving them back a portion of their own earnings in the shape of alms.[72]

Fear must have had a part in middle-class motivation but it did not dominate their actions. The comforting stereotype of the cholera victim stayed with them to the end. When cholera came it was concentrated in the poorer areas of the large towns, and the occasional case in the better areas did not break the impression of safety. The experience of young Henry Solly must have represented many middle-class memories of the first epidemic.

One morning in the summer of 1832, he paid a call at his father's house in St Mary Axe, on his way to his shipping agency office in Leadenhall Street, when he found two clerks guarding the door and forbidding entry. There had been many cases of cholera in London in the previous few weeks –

> but its presence in our midst did not cause any particular alarm either to the circle in which I lived or to myself – it did not seem to concern us at all, and it was with simply a feeling of surprise that I learnt from the clerks on the steps that a young medical man, a pupil of my brother's, who was just going on a distant voyage as the ship's

doctor, had been taken ill of cholera in my brother's rooms and died there in the course of a few hours...

This melancholy catastrophe brought home to us the reality of the visitation, yet I can't remember feeling any anxiety or seeing others terrified.[73]

Cholera had been anticipated with terror and foreboding but when it came there was curiously little panic and disorganisation.

There was no flight from the cities comparable to the exodus from Defoe's London during the plague. A small and cautious part of the middle class did leave the towns. Greville in London wrote – '...many people have taken flight, and others are suspended between their hopes of safety in the country air and their dread of being removed from metropolitan aid'. Southey was at the receiving end of this migration: 'Keswick is filled with refugees from all these places [places with cholera], great as the improbability of our escape is...'[74] Ascribing all this exodus to cholera was an illusion, for the wealthier portions of urban society had been leaving town during the summer in increasing numbers to seek the healthier environment of country estates and spa watering places. In 1832, cholera was doubtless much talked of, among the social and health reasons which took society to Bath, Harrogate, Buxton and Keswick. Many doctors mentioned the fear and anxiety among their patients and blamed the Press and the handbills for this. The nervousness was clear from rumours like the one which suggested that Mrs D. of Belgrave Square had died of fright during the London epidemic. A portion of the middle class fled from the towns but they did that anyway in the summer. There was nothing to compare with the 700 per day who left Paris at the peak of the epidemic or the 50,000 who left Moscow when cholera approached.[75]

Cholera in Britain did not disrupt life on the scale seen in Astrakhan where commercial life had ground to a halt. The trade slump was blamed on cholera, but overproduction and quarantine regulations were more likely causes. Only in the disaster villages where a small community was hit by an explosive epidemic did cholera bring life to a halt. The Staffordshire iron manufacturing and coal mining town of Bilston came close to paralysis as the death toll neared 50 at the end of August:

To describe the consternation of the people is impossible. Manufactories and workshops are closed; business completely at a stand; women seen in a state of distraction running in all directions

for medical help for dying husbands, husbands for their wives, and
children for their parents; the hearse carrying the dead to the grave
without intermission either by day or night. Those inhabitants who
possessed the means of quitting their homes, flying to some purer
atmosphere; those who remained seeing nothing before them but
disease and death. . . .

When community life did come near to breakdown, it was the middle
class who left. In August many of the respectable inhabitants of Bilston
had left and several manufactories were closed as a consequence. Parson
Leigh noted that it was the private pews in the church which were
empty.[76] The small villages of Scotland were the most vulnerable to
disorganisation. When Aberdeen surgeon John Paterson was sent to the
nearby fishing villages of Footdee and Collieston, he found:

All work was suspended; since, indeed, the villagers had been
prevented by the public authorities from entering the towns with
their fish for sale. Thus immured in their small and dirty hovels, all
mental and physical energy forsook them. . . .[77]

Dumfries was the only large settlement in Britain which reported major
signs of panic. When Edward Alison arrived from Edinburgh to help the
hard-pressed local doctors, he found:

Previous to my attendance on the Board, I observed that the greater
number of the shops were shut, the streets covered and spread with
quicklime, the hearse slowly traversing the various lanes and followed
by the nearest relatives of the deceased. . .The panic was so great that
several thousand persons fled and during several days, all of which
time nearly, the rain fell in torrents, scarcely an individual was met
with in the street — the medical men's gigs and the hearse only were
heard. . .[78]

Except for Bilston, no other British town with a population of over
10,000 had a death rate greater than Dumfries with 3.6 per cent. The
Lancet survey suggested that the small towns and villages of Scotland
and Ireland were more liable to panic in response to cholera than those
in England. This may have arisen from a different understanding of the
nature of cholera or from the simpler nature of the economies of these
settlements which made flight less costly in economic terms.[79]

This lack of major panic or disorganisation in the face of cholera was another indication of the basic stability of British society. Bilston was an exception which showed what might have happened if society had been disrupted by cholera. Many of the middle class left, local rates and voluntary subscriptions were inadequate, even the supply of coffins ran out, but the evangelical parson, sure of his faith, remained as one source of leadership. Subscriptions came from all over the country, and the coffins were imported to be rather tactlessly stacked against the wall of the cholera hospital. Places like Leeds and Oxford were more typical. Men like James Montgomery and Henry Solly were representative of middle-class behaviour. In part they were held by the aristocratic concept of duty. In part, the logic of an industrial economy, more fully developed than in France or Russia, held the middle class to their offices and counting houses to ensure their profits and incomes. The development of industrial society was also separating out the British middle class in suburbs like the Park Estate in Leeds and the New Town in Edinburgh. In these new developments, physically separate from the disease threat of the lower classes of society, the middle class were more prepared to stay and take their place as leaders of the community.

During the Reform Bill agitation of 1832, the middle classes of most British towns behaved in a manner which was uniform, consistent and showed that the disregard for the dangers of cholera was not restricted to individuals. Despite Board of Health warnings against large gatherings and contact with infected people and places, the middle class organised a series of major public meetings to press for reform of Parliament just as the cholera began its spread in April and May 1832. The cholera came to London in March just as the third Reform Bill was sent to the Lords. On 8 May, the crisis reached its height. The Lords rejected the Bill. Lord Grey's Whig government resigned. On 15 May, Grey was recalled as Prime Minister, and on 4 June the Bill passed its third reading in the House of Lords. Throughout the crisis, the Reform Bill was supported by mass meetings in all parts of the country. The challenge to the established constitution by the wide-ranging alliance of Whig aristocrats, urban leaders, and middle- and working-class radicals was sustained throughout the days of May. Far from cholera diverting attention from the Reform Bill as the working-class radicals claimed, the Reform Bill diverted attention from cholera. There was a large meeting at Greenock on 1 May, although 154 had already died of cholera. On 11 May, the electors of Westminster met to hear Sir Francis Burdett at the Crown and Anchor Tavern, when Westminster already had 40 dead and London over 900. Cholera was declared in Liverpool on the 12th, and on the 14th the respectable inhabitants attended a meeting in support of the

Class, Power and Cholera   125

Bill addressed by the leading citizens, Brocklebanks, Roscoes and Rathbones. On the 12th, 70,000 gathered on Glasgow Green, as the death toll neared 500. In Leeds, 50,000 met in the Cloth Hall Yard as cholera moved up the Ouse. Birmingham, Derby, Dundee, Manchester, even Newcastle, Darlington and Gateshead, recovering from the winter epidemic, all held meetings as did many more places. Cholera did nothing to deter large numbers of the middle and working classes from these huge gatherings. There were isolated signs of nervousness. Travellers to the Reform Meeting at Cromarty were smoked with sulphur before being allowed in, but for most people politics had priority over health.[80] Although observers as varied as Kay and Cobbett commented on middle-class fears of cholera and fears of the working classes who brought cholera, there was little evidence of this fear in May and June, for the middle-class leadership gathered their own class, and large numbers of the working classes they were supposed to fear, in mass meetings of 30,000 to 70,000 at a time.

(vi) Stability

Inequality in itself is a source of tension between classes as it is between individuals, but a far more potent source of conflict and dynamic change in relationships between groups are the disappointed expectations which one class may hold about the other. This was the case in the cholera epidemic of 1832. No one rose to complain of the differential in class-specific death rate as they rose to challenge the parliamentary franchise. The middle and ruling class saw cholera as a massive threat to the social and economic well-being of the community on which their prosperity depended, and they reacted sharply to that threat. Their reactions with its regulations and hospitals broke the 'rules' of stable class relationships, rules which gave an unstable legitimacy to inequality. Such a breach brought a violent reaction and the traditional respect for the recognised freedoms of the poor was quickly restored. This freedom was only the freedom to die and be buried in peace, if it clashed with more modern values which demanded the maximum use of scientific knowledge to protect life, no matter. The middle class showed little evidence of panic. They stayed in the cholera towns and operated the social and administrative institutions which were part of their claims to power. Despite the tension brought by cholera and the violent popular rejection of some of the administrative solutions, British society, in the short run, returned rapidly to stable equilibrium. As a source of change, cholera in 1832 operated in the longer term. A small section of the middle class, mainly doctors, were dissatisfied with the failure to achieve the aims of the new science-based humanitarian values which wanted to stop cholera, not just to deal with the damage done by the disease. Their reaction was part of the epilogue to 1832.

Notes

1. P. Hollis, *The Pauper Press*, Oxford, 1970; J.H. Wiener, *The War of the Unstamped*, New York, 1969.
2. The ballad is in the British Museum.
3. *Cobbett's Weekly Political Register*, vol.75, 25 February 1832.
4. *The Loyal Reformer's Gazette*, Glasgow, 31 March, 16 April and 28 April 1832.
5. *Times*, 16 February 1832.
6. *Poor Man's Advocate*, no.6, 25 February 1832; *Carpenter's Political Magazine*, Part II, 1831-2, p.49.
7. *Lancet*, 10 December 1832.
8. John Warter Wood (ed.), *Selections from the Letters of Robert Southey*, 4 vols., London, 1856, vol.iv, p.230; *The British Critic*, vol.11, 1832, p.382; *The Christian Observer*, vol.32, 1832, p.125.
9. *New Monthly Magazine*, vol.31, 1831, p.490.
10. L.T. Jennings, *The Correspondence and Diaries of the late Rt. Hon. John Wilson Croker*, 3 vols., London, 1884, vol.ii, p.149; See, for example, *Carpenter's Political Magazine*, vol.1, February 1832.
11. *Poor Man's Advocate*, no.26, 14 July 1832.
12. *The Wesleyan Methodist Magazine*, 1832, p.449.
13. *Poor Man's Advocate*, no.28, 28 July 1832.
14. William Lovett, *Life and Struggles*, London, 1876, p.78.
15. *Loyal Reformer's Gazette*, 4 February and 3 March 1832.
16. Hubert Cole, *Things for the Surgeon*, London, 1964; C. Newman, *The Evolution of Medical Education in the 19th Century*, London, 1957; *S.C. on the Improvement of Health of Towns: Internment of Bodies*, P.P. (H. of C.), vol.X, 1842.
17. *Hansard's Parliamentary Debates*, new series, vols. 18-20, 29 January 1828 – 30 March 1829 and vol.21, 5 May 1829; *S.C. on Anatomy*, P.P. (H. of C.), vol.VII, 1828.
18. *Westminster Review*, vol.10, 1828-9, p.128.
19. Hospital Returns, London, April 1832, P.R.O., P.C.1/111. Robert Christison, 'Account of the arrangements made by the Edinburgh Board of Health preparatory to the arrival of cholera in that city', *E.M.S.J.*, vol.37, 1832, p.cclxviii.
20. Henry Gaulter, *The Origins and Progress of the Malignant Cholera in Manchester...*, London, 1833, p.138.
21. *Poor Man's Advocate*, no.26, 14 July 1832; *Cobbett's Political Register*, vol.76, 7 April 1832; Post-Mortem Reports, P.R.O., P.C.1/103.
22. Gaulter, *Malignant Cholera in Manchester*, p.138.
23. Oxford Board of Health Minute Book, *loc. cit.*, 11 July 1832.
24. W. Haslewood and W. Mordey, *The History and Medical Treatment of Cholera as it appeared in Sunderland in 1831*, London, 1832, p.132; George W. Baker and Dwight W. Chapman (eds.), *Man and Society in Disaster*, New York, 1962, pp.12 and 185-299.
25. From St Anne's, Middlesex, 13 February 1832, P.R.O., P.C.1/103; *S.C. on Internment*, P.P. (H. of C.), 1842, vol.X, Q.613 and 1974-1980.
26. George Watt, 'On the Origin and Spread of Malignant Cholera in Glasgow and

its Neighbourhood', *Glasgow Medical Journal*, vol.5, 1832, p.384; *S.C. on the Improvement of Health of Towns*, loc. cit. Q.683.
27. Rev. W. Leigh, *An Authentic Narrative of the Melancholy Occurrences at Bilston... during the Awful Visitation in that Town of Cholera...*, Wolverhampton, 1833, pp.39-40.
28. Thomas Shapter, *The History of Cholera in Exeter*, London, 1849, pp.142-76; Hubert Cole, *Things for the Surgeon*, p.161.
29. *Jackson's Oxford Journal*, 28 July 1832.
30. *Poor Man's Guardian*, no.66, 15 September 1832.
31. *John Bull*, 16 January 1832; *The Cholera Gazette*, no.1, 14 January 1832.
32. *Lancet*, 1832, vol.II, p.74; *E.M.S.J.*, vol.36, 1831, p.122; Review and Quotation from D.J.R. Lichtenstadt, *Die Asiatic Cholera in Russland...*, Berlin, 1831; also quoted in *Westminster Review*, vol.15, 1831, p.470.
33. *Cobbett's Political Register*, vol.74, 10 December 1831.
34. *Poor Man's Advocate*, no.32, 25 April 1832.
35. Oxford Board of Health, General Account Book, Bodleian Library Oxford, MSS. Top Oxon c.270.
36. Henry Pelling, *Popular Politics and Society in Late Victorian Britain*, London, 1968.
37. *Hansard's Parliamentary Debates*, 3rd series, vol.11, 28 March 1832.
38. *Standard*, 30 March 1832.
39. *Edinburgh Evening Courant*, 17 March 1832.
40. *Glasgow Courier*, 17 March 1832; *Glasgow Chronicle*, 16 March 1832.
41. *Glasgow Courier*, 27 March 1832; *Glasgow Chronicle*, 26 March 1832; *The Loyal Reformer's Gazette*, 24 March 1832.
42. *Glasgow Chronicle*, 30 March 1832.
43. *Times*, 4 September 1832; *Standard*, 4 September 1832; *John Bull*, 10 September 1832.
44. J.P. Kay, *The Moral and Physical Condition of the Working Classes...*, Manchester, 1832, pp.36-40.
45. *Poor Man's Advocate*, 31 March, 25 April and 28 July 1832.
46. *Poor Man's Advocate*, 15 September 1832.
47. 'Cholera – Ignorance and Knowledge', *Phrenological Journal*, vol.7, 1831-2, p.463.
48. *Hansard's Parliamentary Debates*, 3rd series, vol.9, 15 December 1831; Fraser Brockington, 'Public Health at the Privy Council, 1831-1834', *Journal of the History of Medicine*, 1961, pp.161-85.
49. Central Board of Health letter book, 13 June 1832, P.R.O., P.C.1/95.
50. W. Reid Clanny, *Cholera in Sunderland*, pp.31-42; W. Haslewood and W. Mordey, *History and Medical Treatment of Cholera*, p.120; Minute Book of the Oxford Board of Health, 18 August 1832, Bodleian Library Oxford, MSS. Top Oxon c.272; Central Board of Health letter book, 22 November 1831, P.R.O., P.C.1/93.
51. Oxford Board of Health Minute Book, 11 July 1832, loc. cit.; *Hansard's Parliamentary Debates*, 3rd series, vol.10, 14 February 1832.
52. E.P. Thompson, 'The Moral Economy of the English Crowd', *Past and Present*, no.50, 1971, pp. 95-116; R.B. Rose, '18th century Price Riots and Public Policy in England', *International Review of Social History*, 1961; George Rudé, *The Crowd in History, 1730-1848*, New York, 1964; E.J. Hobsbawm and George Rudé, *Captain Swing*, London, 1969.
53. Robert Christison, *E.M.S.J.*, vol.37, 1832.
54. The handbills discussed so far are in the archives of the Radcliffe Infirmary, Oxford and the local history collection in Oxford City Libraries.
55. Thomas Wilson Collection, vol.3, f.750-55, Newcastle-upon-Tyne Central Library.

56. Henry Gaulter, *Malignant Cholera in Manchester*, p.137.
57. R.K. Webb, 'Working Class Readers in Early Victorian England', *English Historical Review*, vol.65, 1950, pp.333-51; and 'Literacy among the Working Classes in 19th Century Scotland', *Scottish Historical Review*, vol.34, 1954, pp.100-14.
58. H.P. Tait, 'The Cholera Board of Health, Edinburgh 1831-1834', *The Medical Officer*, vol.98, 25 October 1957.
59. A. Briggs, 'The Background of the Parliamentary Reform Movement in three English Cities, 1830-1832', *Cambridge Historical Journal*, vol.X, 1952; *Leeds Mercury*, 27 June 1835, for a survey of the Old Corporation.
60. Oxford Board of Health Minute Book, loc. cit., 11 July 1832.
61. See previous chapters and Gwen Hart, *A History of Cheltenham*, Leicester, 1965, p.283; Account Book of the Liberton Board of Health, Scottish Record Office, CH 2/383 30; *The Cholera Gazette*, 28 January 1832.
62. *Directions to plain people as a guide to their conduct during the cholera*, London, 1831.
63. Rough note, 10 January 1832, agreeing to put a notice to this effect in the North of England newspapers, P.R.O., P.C.1/111.
64. *Cholera Gazette*, 28 January 1832.
65. George Watt, *Glasgow Medical Journal*, vol.5, 1832.
66. Rev. W. Leigh, *Occurrences at Bilston*; *Wesleyan Methodist Magazine*, 1832, p.748.
67. *Hansard's Parliamentary Debates*, 3rd series, vol.9, 15 December 1831; J.W. Wood, *Letters of Robert Southey*, vol.iv, p.249; John Holland and James Everett, *Memoirs of James Montgomery*, 7 vols., London, 1856, vol.5, p.54.
68. *Monthly Review*, vol.3, 1831.
69. *New Monthly Magazine*, vol.31, 1831, p.526.
70. *Cobbett's Weekly Political Register*, vol.75, 26 February 1832.
71. *Poor Man's Guardian*, 19 November 1831 and 18 February 1832.
72. *Poor Man's Advocate*, 3 March 1832.
73. Henry Solly, *These Eighty Years*, 2 vols., London, 1893.
74. *The Greville Papers*. vol.ii, p.316, 25 July 1832; J.W. Wood, *Letters of Robert Southey*, vol.iv, p.293.
75. L. Chevalier, *Le Choléra*, Paris. 1958; R.E. McGrew. *Russia and the Cholera, 1823-32*, Madison, 1965.
76. *The Standard*, 30 August 1832; Rev. W. Leigh, *Occurrences at Bilston*, pp.41-3.
77. John Paterson, 'Observations on the Cholera as it appeared at Collieston and Footdee, Aberdeenshire', *E.M.S.J.*, vol.49, 1838, pp.408-12.
78. Edward Alison, Edinburgh to Mr. McLean, 21 November 1832, P.R.O., P.C.1/103; this report is confirmed by *A short account of the origin and progress of the Cholera Morbus, particularly its ravages in Dumfries in September, October and November 1832*, by a Citizen, Dumfries, 1833. A closer study of this remarkable epidemic may well suggest reasons for the greater alarm felt in Scotland.
79. *Lancet*, vol.I, 1833, p.203. He mentions Sligo and Enniskillen as the places worst affected.
80. *Times*, 1-14 May 1832; Peter MacKenzie, *Reminiscences of Glasgow and the West of Scotland*, Glasgow, 1866, vol.ii, p.340; *Leeds Mercury*, 12 May, 15 May and 16 June 1832; Hugh Miller, *My Schools and Schoolmasters*, pp.483-91.

7 RELIGION AND MORALS

Religion and morality were central to British society's reaction to the cholera of 1831 and 1832. Historians of disease and public health tend to concentrate on the pre-history of our own modes of thought and action, the miasma-contagion disputes, the problems of administration and finance and the campaign to gain political support for reform. This neglects the part which moral and metaphysical ideas played in the response to cholera and other diseases. Witches, spirits and gods are easily accepted as part of the thinking of the Nuer tribes of East Africa or even the Englishmen of the sixteenth and seventeenth centuries, when they faced disease and ill fortune.[1] The people of the industrial revolution are so like ourselves in many of their habits and thought patterns that such aspects of their reaction to events are often ignored or derided as 'fatalism'. There is a basic human need to impose a pattern on events so that these may be explained, judged and perhaps controlled. Morality, religion, social structure, scientific understanding and material culture, all limit and influence these patterns. The need became even greater when events involved the pain and suffering brought by cholera. In the face of this terrible and inexplicable threat individuals needed some guide which would enable them to carry on their lives with reasonable calm and order; governments needed some imperative which would gain the co-operation of their subjects in measures to combat the threat. Science could not provide this certainty.[2] Science was unconvincing and would persuade no one of the value of public health measures. Therefore religious and moral explanations and imperatives played a greater part than in later industrial society.

The relationship between God and cholera was not a simple one. Few men denied Providence some part in the causes of the epidemic. Most had their Bible and a chosen cholera medicine on the shelf. Working out the details of the relationship was left to the clergy and ministers of the various sects and churches of Britain, who pressed their views on government and people through sermons, pamphlets and periodicals. The religious divisions of England and Scotland were important not only because they reflected differences in theology and church government, but also because each church and sect tended to represent different social and economic groups and different views on the proper structure of society.[3] These social perspectives were as crucial as theological ones for the formation of the religious explanations of cholera. In many cases the language of religion was a code which enabled many groups to express social anxieties which were highlighted by cholera.

Cholera came as the hundred-year truce between religion and science was drawing to a close. Descartes had neatly separated the world of the mind and the soul from the physical world and enabled churchmen and scientists to make their slow way through the eighteenth century without conflict. The early nineteenth-century attacks upon religion had little to do with science and rarely approached atheism. The established church was seen as the supporter of social injustice, with its clerical magistrates, game laws, repression of radicals and their political views, the rejection of the Reform Bill in 1832 by the bishops in the House of Lords, and the general indifference of the church to poverty. The Bible was displayed as a catalogue of moral and logical inconsistencies. Paine, Hone, Carlile, Owen and Holyoake all attacked Christianity on moral and social grounds; intellectual argument followed later to justify belief in unbelief.[4]

It was another generation before Darwin and Huxley brought science and religion into direct conflict, before scientific method with its demands for evidence and proof destroyed the supernatural world of the spirit and thus Christ's whole mission of salvation. In 1832, it was geology which proved the most radical and subversive challenge to religion and those who based their faith on the literal acceptance of the Bible as the word of God. The issues, the progress and the opposing viewpoints of the religious debate over geological discovery were very similar to those of the religious discussion of cholera. Hutton, Sedgewick and Buckland had revealed a world of extinct volcanoes, of mountain building and folding, of strata packed with fossils of long extinct animals and plants, of strata which took longer than the six days of Genesis to create. Christian thinking responded to this challenge with a fundamental debate about the relationship between God and scientific laws. The debate took place in the context of Archdeacon Paley's views on natural theology. Paley argued that the scientist and the natural theologian were continually revealing the natural laws which maintained man in harmony with nature and sustained God's creation, thus demonstrating the existence of a rational and benevolent God, creator, designer and scientific law-giver. Geology was opportunity and threat to the Christian thinker. The successive strata might be footsteps of the creator, making geology a form of worship, but the threat to Genesis was still present. Some suggested that the 'day' of Genesis might be better translated as a very long time, not just 24 hours. Thomas Chalmers represented most evangelical thinkers when he rejected all this and accepted the six days as 'literally a week of miracles – the period of great creative interposition'. In the absence of Darwinian theories of survival of the fittest and an understanding of mutation, theologians of all varieties were puzzled by the existence of geological strata, each with a totally new series of plants and animals and no apparent link with the previous series. It hardly seemed rational of God to set aside scientific laws once laid down, yet why should there be several periods of 'creative interposition' or miracles, which seemed the only way to account for the new species. Cholera, unpredictable and unexplained, was caught in this pattern of argument. The disease might be the result of purposeful divine intervention, or the result of some secondary cause as yet undiscovered. In the Christian mind the concept of an interventionist God, of an ever watchful and benevolent creator, was being challenged by the more distant rule of God the designer, whose laws were seen through the workings of nature, to guide and be discovered by the human mind.[5]

The most active religious movement which deeply influenced the response to cholera was not identified with any church or chapel organisation. It was a movement which crossed the boundaries of church and denomination, softening some and hardening others. The evangelical founded his faith upon the personal experience of conversion. His faith was gained and sustained by the reading and inspiration of the Bible, by prayer and by good works, and the greatest of all good works was to spread the word of God and seek the conversion of others. It was an emotional movement which pressed those who felt its power into a whole range of social activities, propaganda, charity and missionary work. At one level of society it drew its strength from the bankers and friends of the Clapham sect, men of the highest status among the middle classes, shocked by the corruption, sensuality and passive attitude to religion among the aristocracy, by the cruel and reckless profit-seeking of the new manufacturers, and by the disloyalty and barbaric vice of the lower classes. Lower in the social scale the Methodist preachers led many to ignore the old issues of predestination and free will and to seek personal salvation through prayer and the recognition of their own guilt. At its best the evangelical movement was involved in the abolition of slavery, in the 1833 Factory Acts and countless small acts of charity to the poor. At its worst, it sought to suppress all Sunday entertainment and created a vicious anti-popery movement out of traditional fears and the resentment of Irish immigration.[6]

The evangelicals saw the cholera as a direct result of the will of Providence. Their God was an interventionist God, the God of miracles in the contemporary scientific debate, a God who directed cholera with justice and purpose. The Wesleyans firmly summed up 1832,

> ...if not a sparrow falls to the ground without our Heavenly Father; an event so important as death can in no instance befall intelligent, redeemed and immortal man, but under Divine direction. "The pestilence walketh in darkness, and the arrow flieth by day", but every victim is selected by infinite wisdom, acting under the direction of mercy or of justice, according to the character of the person whose days are numbered.[7]

These ideas were shared by the Congregational and Baptist churches, by the Secession churches of Scotland, as well as the evangelicals of the Kirk and the Anglican church. As men sought to pattern the world with their own desire for morality and justice, such terrible afflictions as cholera could only be seen as a form of punishment. Such punishment could only come as retribution for sin against the wishes of an all-powerful God. Thus pain and death became explicable, legitimate and more bearable.

The relationship between sin and the suffering of individuals was not simple. As the Methodists observed, 'Many burning and shining lights have been quenched in darkness.' They lost many members, elders and ministers. In Newcastle, one Scottish Secession church lost a minister of 'irreproachable' character, but admitted he lived near the cholera hospital. The Auxiliary Tract Society lost one of their distributors in Southwark, a poor but Christian woman. Such losses were accepted with sorrow and the consolation that 'the righteous shall be held in everlasting remembrance', and would achieve salvation through the intervention of Christ.[8]

The deaths of the righteous and the view that cholera was a 'scourge' sent to punish sin were compatible, for the sins might be those of mankind as a species, of the nation of which he was a part, or himself as an individual. The *Christian Observer* reminded its readers that 'the guilt is theirs in common with all the fallen children of Adam'.[9]

For over a generation the evangelical mind had been concerned about national morals and was acutely aware of the link between morals and social order. The years 1831 and 1832 appeared to be years of mounting social, economic and political chaos to which the violence of cholera was a final terrifying addition.

Religion and Morals   133

> To a very great extent, the present is a day of adversity. . . . In such
> times the duty of God's people is plain. 'The Lord's voice crieth
> unto the city'. Public affairs are in a state of extreme agitation —
> commerce, as well as trade of all kinds is at a low ebb — the fatal
> pestilence like a destroying angel, has set its foot upon our shores,
> and pauses only till the Almighty sovereign shall seal its commission
> — infidelity vaunteth itself at the corners of the streets and in the
> markets — violence has been rampant in our cities — wasting and
> destruction have entered into all our borders — the church
> languishes — its vintage faileth — fanaticism and speculation like a
> wrathful bolt from the skies, have scattered some of the Cedars of
> Lebanon — we have seen contention and strife among brethren in
> the city. . . .[10]

A trade slump, the Reform Bill crisis which brought riots and dozens of
threatening and noisy meetings, sectarian disputes, the constant mocking
of the church by men like Carlile and Hone, and the association of such
ideas with the aggressive radicalism of the growing unstamped Press,
together with the Divine warning, cholera, all confirmed the evangelical
belief that decline in morality, especially decline in respect for the
church, would bring social chaos in its wake.

The *Christian Observer* was typical of those who were not very
specific about what the nation had done wrong; 'the widespread
prevalence of infidelity and profaneness', was the only charge they
made.[11] The Methodists were not so vague. Infidelity and sectarian
animosity were high on their list of sins. They especially resented the
established clergy's contempt for dissenters, and went on,

> What Christian can contemplate the excessive intemperance
> prevailing in all classes of society throughout this country and not
> mourn? Who that fears God can witness the desecration of the Holy
> Sabbath by boats, vans and coaches; by the immense issue of
> newspapers; by parties of pleasure and business; and by the
> announcement of cabinet dinners — and not sigh before Him on
> account of these abominations, and tremble while He anticipates the
> consequences?

The Wesleyans were one of the few groups to suggest that 'the
sufferings of the labouring poor in England', especially their inadequate
level of wages, might be a cause of just anger from God, for their
situation was 'such as to seriously interfere with their spiritual interests'.

The extreme Presbyterian *Covenanter* agreed with all this but had a special concern of its own. They had none of the reticence of the English evangelicals who referred indirectly to idolatry and the decline of religion.

Of late years, not only has she [Britain] authoritatively tolerated the idolatry of the east, but on the continent she has been the mainstay of the pillars of antiChrist, and at home the delusions of Popery have received the fullest encouragement.

A glance at the Book of Ezekiel indicated that pestilence was the punishment for those who countenanced idolatry, and few needed reminding that Catholic Emancipation had been granted a few years before.[12]

The sins of Adam and the morals of the nation were important, but the individual who wanted to avoid cholera needed more specific advice on the misdeeds he must avoid to be safe from the wrath of the Lord. The evangelical Anglicans were again vague. They had little more than dire warnings to 'flee from sin, flee from the wrath to come'.[13] Many of the other denominations were prepared to be more specific about sin. One Congregational minister from Sunderland felt that industry was a great moral preventative against threats like cholera and warned 'those who have combined indolence with vice have hitherto been its first victims'.[14] The Methodists were again the most direct about sin. They gave case histories which were as detailed and purposeful as those of the medical journals, although the Methodist and the medical man were informed by completely different principles of explanation in their search for an answer to the threat of cholera. The *Methodist Magazine* surveyed the first cases at Gateshead in exhaustive and exhausting detail,

> On the day following Christmas day two men, one living in the town and the other a few miles in the country, attended a cock fight in the afternoon; and at a public house partook of a supper with the company which had been engaged in this cruel and wicked sport. While at the supper the townsman was seized with cholera, and was a corpse in about twelve hours. The countryman was assailed...as soon as he got home, and within two days was also in eternity.
>
>   A man in —— Bank who was a confirmed drunkard and notorious cockfighter was induced to attend a place of worship on the Sunday evening. What he then heard alarmed his conscience. On

reaching home, he told his wife he 'was in the way to hell', took off the heads of his cocks, and declared he would change his life...he was seized by cholera and permitted to enter the house of God no more! God, however, spared him two days during which he fervently prayed for mercy; and we trust that mercy was granted at this eleventh hour.

A man in Newcastle...a dreadful swearer and notorious Sabbath breaker, as well as a confirmed drunkard, was seized by cholera; whilst in the agonies of death, he called for ardent spirits and died in a few hours.

A female in the higher part of —— was repeatedly reproved for her violation of the holy Sabbath, neglect of public worship, and her horrible practice of swearing...cholera seized her...She entreated her friends to pray for her adding, 'My heart is hard: I cannot feel; I cannot pray. When I might have prayed, and could have prayed I would not. Now I would but cannot!' Without any visible change, she left this world to appear before her judge.

On the Christmas day, two men (one of whom was a notorious dog fighter) were fighting in a public house, in a state of intoxication, near the Wesleyan chapel, and that too during the time of worship there. One of them died of the cholera in a few hours after, and the other in two days!

A backslider, in ——, who had returned to his old crime of intemperance...was seized by this malady in the evening, and was dead before the next morning's light.

O how has this sweeping scourge cut down the ungodly! Some pious souls may have been removed by it, and have spent their last moments in peace; but the dissipated, dissolute, profane, and intemperate, are the general victims of the disease![15]

For the varied and specific way in which they listed sins, the Methodists were unrivalled. The Lord evidently picked his targets with unerring accuracy as the unrepentant sinner was struck down. If the grim and almost savage satisfaction with which this relentless catalogue of sin and death was presented lacked all charity and compassion, it must be remembered it was written by men who had no control over the threat they faced — their feeling of helplessness in the face of cholera was reflected in this lack of charity, for they had no help to offer but the brief chance of repentance.

Of all the sins to which flesh was heir, the abuse of alcoholic drink was the most often mentioned. Drink was crucial to the moral analysis of cholera in Britain, and featured in many explanations which had no mention of God or morality. When observers began to generalise about the personal habits which made one man rather than another liable to the terrifying disaster of a cholera attack, their attention was inevitably drawn to his drinking habits. In 1832, Britain was an alcohol-using society which was just beginning to question the uncritical acceptance of all the evils, pleasures and relaxation which drink had brought to so many generations. Drink was so closely bound in with so many social relationships that few men could have avoided its frequent use in situations of varied importance in their life and fortune.

Drink was the basis of friendship and conversation. For the working classes in the crowded one-room, one-family tenements and the back-to-backs of the growing towns, the public house served the function of sitting room, as well as being the provider of companionship, newspapers, entertainment and even insurance in the form of the Friendly Society. Drink eased the path of courtship and sealed business agreements. It was energy and payment for workers in the fields, in ironworks, in the London docks and on the keels of the Tyne. It was warmth for travellers, comfort for the sick and a valuable ally for those facing the surgeon's knife.

The generation which faced cholera was one which was beginning to reassess the place of drink in society. The standard of living of the middle class had made steady progress since the beginning of the century. Their homes were better furnished and more comfortable. Thus they came to drink less at the Inn and more at home entertaining friends for dinner parties and soirées, attended by their servants. Thus public drunkenness and, by association, drink itself became a sign of low social status. This trend of opinion was supported by the views of the evangelicals. They saw drink as sensual indulgence, a barrier between God and man, an impediment to conversion as well as a source of improvident social irresponsibility. Such changes in opinion are slow but if a date had to be found at which drinking was dropped from the behaviour pattern of the respectable middle class, that date would be somewhere near 1832. The first temperance societies were founded in 1831, pledging their members to the moderate use of beer and wine and abstinence from spirits. In 1833, *Pickwick Papers* was published, the last major British novel to portray drunkenness as acceptable, jolly, Christmas-style fun. Thus, by 1832, drink and moral judgement had become associated in several different and related ways. A man's character could still be judged by the way he behaved in drinking situations. Increasingly, nineteenth-century society saw that his status

Religion and Morals 137

and wealth was indicated by the way he drank. Then the morality of drink itself was questioned as alcohol was linked directly with poverty, with neglect of religion and with the loss of personal respect and independence.[16]

Cholera and drink rapidly became associated. Drink had a central place in the stereotype of a cholera victim created by the early case reports and this continued throughout the epidemic,

> He was a cobbler by trade, and one of those reprobates whom cholera is said to know for its victims — an idle, quarrelsome, profane drunkard, starving both himself and his family.

This Manchester man had recently been injured in a fight and cholera took him whilst he was drunk.[17]

The same advice came from all shades of opinion and all sorts and conditions of men — avoid alcoholic drink, or at least use it in moderation. The Central Board of Health, the middle-class periodicals and the radical unstamped Press, all repeated the same message. *Directions to Plain People* advised, 'Use wine in moderation, but drink no spirituous liquors, and indulge in no irregular and vicious habits, for these materially increase the virulence of cholera.' This advice was very close in its wording to the moderationist pledge of the early temperance societies.[18] They were naturally delighted with the advice which the government gave. The Black Country parsons, Girdlestone and Leigh both saw the link between drink and cholera as part of God's punishment of sinners. Christmas Day in Gateshead was a terrible example of 'God's judgement'.

> About noon on Christmas Day (which was also the Holy Sabbath) in the lower part of this town, and in Bottle Bank, such scenes of drunkenness and outrage were witnessed, as would be disgraceful in a heathen country. Men and women were staggering in a state of complete intoxication. Some were brawling and fighting, while crowds were collected as spectators of their shame. The streets in this case were almost impassable. 'But because of these things the wrath of God cometh upon the children of disobedience'. That night and the following days awefully verified this divinely inspired declaration.

By 5 January there were 102 dead in Gateshead, one of the most savage outbreaks of the epidemic.[19]

This advice and association would have been easily accepted by many people for they already associated drink with many minor and major personal disasters. Although the idea was developed by administrative, medical and religious sections of the middle and upper classes, it was readily adopted by the working-class Press. This was not surprising, for the radical leadership whose ideas were reflected in this Press were soon to make temperance, especially its extremist form, teetotalism, a part of their claim to independence, respectability and political rights. Under the pressure of the fears brought by cholera, the extreme development of a changing moral viewpoint was presented as a widely applicable medical and public health measure.

The link between drink and cholera was confirmed by many empirical observations made during the epidemic. There was a negative correlation between drink and cholera if they were taken in isolation. The brewery workers of Edinburgh, Glasgow and many parts of London escaped the epidemic.[20] They lived in heavily infected areas, but had a steady supply of beer from their employers and thus rarely touched the water supplies which spread the disease. But drink was part of a social and environmental complex of poverty, deprivation and disease, such as George Watt saw in the Goosedubs area of Glasgow,

> ...its inhabitants (from 8,000 to 10,000) of the most destitute class, ill fed, ill clothed, ill lodged, (often scarcely a bundle of straw for a bed, without a single covering) and I may add too often most intemperate in their habits, converting every valuable they possess, into money, to procure spirits, or spending what money they earn or receive from charitable funds in the same manner.[21]

In such areas with inadequate water supplies, usually wells, and no sanitation, overflowing privy middens seeped into the wells, and heavy drinking could have a strong positive correlation with cholera.

The men of 1832 could not have known that there was a sound physiological basis for the empirical and moral judgements they made about drink and cholera. Although healthy people are not safe, they do survive quite heavy doses of infection without developing cholera. The *vibrio* is often destroyed by the acids of the mouth or stomach before it can reach the favourable alkaline environment of the stomach where it will thrive. Chronic gastritis, and many irregularities and disorders of the stomach are frequently the lot of those who habitually abuse alcohol. These stomach upsets allow the *vibrio* to escape the action of stomach acids, and thus the drunkard is and was more liable to develop cholera than the sober person. Besides, this heavy drinking and the malnutrition which accompanied it predisposed to a wide range of infections, including cholera. There was a congruence here between moral, social and scientific judgement which would have delighted the natural theologian as proof that the will of God was carried out in the physiology of the human body. On the other hand the moderate use of alcohol stimulates the stomach acids so the careful drinker will be better protected than the abstainer.[22]

For the evangelical, the cholera epidemic was a massive demonstration of the power of God. The epidemic showed 'how completely are life and health and all things in the hands of God'.[23] This demonstration had a double purpose.

Cholera was sent to confound the 'pride', 'the impotent boastings of modern science...in these days of medical skill and rational habits'.[24] The Congregational Minister from Sunderland considered that when science reached perfection it would once again conform to scriptural Christianity. The present conflict was caused by the 'cold and dreary materialism' of the men who were investigating scientific laws, who ignored 'the principles of God's moral government'. Cholera asserted the superiority of religion over science; 'the stroke of this messenger of God is upon intellectual deities, the gods of philosophical idolatry, as well as upon the grosser vices of the vulgar.'[25] This scarce-concealed exultation over the defeat of science spelt future trouble for religious consciousness in Britain. If the authority of God was to depend upon the continued failure of science, then the foundations of faith were indeed vulnerable.

Yet in his defence of an all powerful and interventionist God, the evangelical was compelled to assert the superiority of religion over science. From his conversion experience and close Bible study and prayer the evangelical had forged a satisfying and direct relationship with his God, and was confident that rewards and punishments would be justly distributed. He was naturally alarmed at the prospect of scientific laws forming a total and impenetrable barrier between God and the believer. A direct clash between science and religion is never necessary, but in practice was and is difficult to avoid for both these aspects of human experience attempt the same task. They take the realities of sense experience and translate them into intelligible language; 'the attempt is made by both to connect things with each other, to establish internal relationships between them, to classify them and to systematise them.'[26]

The classifications, systems and causal relationships of religion and science tend to diverge, for religion endows them with divine purpose.

God is eternal, purposefully uniting moral and physical laws and events, whilst science seeks out observed regularities as a basis for prediction and decision and reserves the right to subject its laws to perpetual criticism and change, thus challenging the eternal stability of religion. Science was an irresponsible and destabilising agent. To the evangelical looking for personal and social stability in a world increasingly threatened by chaos, science was a threat to be countered.

Cholera, which could strike down a healthy man without warning in a few hours, was more than this. It was a reminder of the frailty of man and the power of God, a call to prayer, repentance and faith, an offer of the salvation of Christ and a terror that would turn men to their religion. Congregationalists, Methodists and Anglicans alike were reminded that 'in the midst of life we are in death'.[27] The experience of death was crucial for the evangelical. It was not only the basis for terrifying sermons and the intense records of countless death-bed scenes which the nineteenth century published or pushed away in many bundles of family papers. Death, which provided the need for eternity, was also the proof that such eternity existed, and the death-bed scenes provided clear proof that all the evangelical teaching about faith and morals was justified, for at the moment of death the evangelical experienced, unfettered by temporal concerns, that direct and personal relationship with his God for which his religious teachings had prepared him. It was natural then that evangelicals — Anglican, Independent and Methodist — should have been most impressed and were most eloquent on the terrifying death scenes which cholera presented.

All religions offer means to salvation — salvation from the day-to-day ills and tensions of the world, from social oppression and degradation, as well as a solution to the greater problems of life after death. Cholera aroused fears at all these levels of human experience. Salvation was the sacred equivalent of the medical man's cure. It required its own régime and treatment — prayer, Bible reading and faith. In many ways religion provided a clearer analysis of cholera than the medical world. Methodists and Presbyterians promised that 'sincere repentance' and prayer would 'stay the Lord's hand'.[28] Girdlestone, in a monumental terror sermon at Sedgely, put the message clearly,

> Which of you can deny that you are for your sins worthy of death; aye, worthy of death eternal? And if of death eternal what is death such as sickness ends in? The struggle of an hour, say a day, what is this to the agony of eternity? And though that agony were not to begin for many years to come, what are years? What, when they

shall have passed, will they seem, compared with ever-lasting destruction? Oh then, if you fear eternal death, oh flee from sin, flee from the wrath to come. Let disease remind you of the sickness of the soul. Let the grave suggest to you the bottomless pit. If you would escape either let no one day more be wasted; repent, amend, obey; in one word, believe.[29]

And so he goes on. Hardly 'comfortable words' in the circumstances.

In a rather calmer mood, the *Congregational Magazine* provided its readers with an article 'Moral Preservatives against Cholera', which included temperance, cleanliness, hard work, fortitude and gospel reading.[30] There was little fatalism in these exhortations to prayer for they were usually accompanied by the best practical advice available. 'The Christian is a citizen, and must sustain his part in every national emergency,' advised the *Evangelical Magazine*. Attention to clothing, food, cholera hospitals, cleanliness and avoiding contagion were needed as well as 'preventative remedies for the soul'. The Kirk said that it was the will of God that men should look for the best cures available and the *Covenanter* helped with copies of the regulations issued by the Boards of Health in Belfast and Edinburgh.[31]

It was natural that a society dominated by Protestant thought gave an important place to Bible reading among spiritual aids during the epidemic. In November, the General Purposes Committee of the British and Foreign Bible Society recommended that the Society should make a loan stock of New Testaments available to their branches and auxiliaries to ensure that no family was without a copy when cholera came, for,

> the truths of the sacred volume, when accompanied by Divine teaching, can minister patience and strong consolation under the severest sufferings, and prepare the immortal spirit for its departure to another world.

By the end of 1832, 19,537 testaments had been distributed. This operation showed the evangelicals at their best and worst. It was a genuine attempt to bring help and comfort, but the editors of the *Missionary Register* could not help noting that it was the Roman Catholic poor who most needed help from the tract distributors of Southwark, and many of the Society's committee-men clearly saw the fear produced by the epidemic as an opportunity to promote their own beliefs. As cholera spread in the Black Country, the district committee of the SPCK decided (my italics) 'that so *excellent* an opportunity ought, by no means, to be lost, for sowing in this method the seed of the gospel'.[32]

It was the Unitarians who defended God the scientist and attacked the evangelical view of the efficacy of prayer,

> Prayers like the confessions of murderers, acknowledging fallacious sins and blinking real crimes, and ascribing human calamities to Divine vindictiveness, are not the means to be employed. We should be up and doing. Every rational effort should be made to grapple with the evils of ignorance and poverty. For this purpose the associating principle should be called into full operation. Every facility should be given for the diffusion of full information.

The Unitarians rejected the notion of direct intervention by God and claimed that God worked by scientific laws which were ascertainable by man. Hence, prayer and fasting could not avert cholera, nor could cholera be punishment for sin, for it 'knows nothing of saint or sinner'. Such ideas denied 'the universality of Providence' for they ignored many other kinds of suffering. Cholera obeyed the fixed laws of physical existence; 'we know that these laws are the universal operations of Providence; hence every suffering is Providential infliction, as every blessing is Providential bounty. . . .' The only sin which cholera exploited was 'the condition of the lower classes' which was 'an invitation to disease' and a result of neglect by the wealthy.

> The efficacy of prayer is not in changing the course of nature. Since the age of miracles its force has never been physical but moral, it is the devout expression of our wishes, but can never effect the accomplishment of our wishes if they be inconsistent with those laws of nature which are the will of God. It may heal the wounded spirit but not the maimed body. It may purify the heart but not the atmosphere. . .[33]

Unitarianism expected no dramatic intervention or miracle. Mankind was expected to use his senses and reason and not take false comfort in prayer and humiliation. Although the Unitarian analysis seems to a modern mind to be very relevant to the problems of 1832, its great flaw was the social aloofness and intellectual coldness of its holders. Unitarianism was the faith of an élite 'out-group' amongst the middle classes — merchants and professional men, divorced from national and often local power – suspected by the majority of the ruling classes, and out of contact with the rest of the population. Unitarianism remained an austere faith, never willing to propagandise itself with the enthusiasm of the evangelical or the scornful fervour of the working-class radical deist. It was an undercurrent which informed many reflective views on the relationship between religion and science, but Unitarians failed to give direct or powerful guidance to the development of religious consciousness in Britain. If their views had achieved a more dominant place, the traumatic clashes later in the century might have been avoided.

Few articulate Christians agreed with the Unitarian view on prayer. Prayer invited the direct intervention of God. The debate over miracles was not just an academic debate on the metaphysics of geology but involved everyday questions of prayer, disease and death. There was ample evidence that prayers had been answered. As the Methodists observed at the end of 1832; 'the dreaded pestilence has almost entirely disappeared'.[34] Besides, cholera had not been as bad as anticipated and not as bad as it had been in an irreligious country like France. When the Wesleyan conference met in Liverpool at the height of the local epidemic the members met with the congregation of Brunswick Chapel for a day of humiliation and prayer. From that day onwards the epidemic died down; 'Whatever sceptics may say, it is no vain thing to call upon the Lord.'[35] Some claims for the success of prayer were a little ill-timed. The *Christian Observer* felt that the epidemic moderated in March 1832 in response to prayer; they were undismayed by the explosive spread of the disease at mid summer and explained that this was a masterly way of confounding the boastings of science. The influence of prayer upon events was and is always debatable. Apparent failure can always be attributed to the inadequacy of the supplicant, success can be written off as something that would have happened in any case (as the Unitarians claimed). The efficacy of prayer was asserted, not proved, one either believed or did not. In any case, in the then state of medical knowledge it was probable that prayer was the most effective preventative which the individual had available to him.

Medical opinion affirmed the value of prayer in at least one respect. The medical men emphasised the value of a calm and tranquil mind as a means of reducing the chances of infection. The evangelicals were sure that prayer was the ideal means of achieving this calm,

> 'the peace of God which passeth all understanding' [will] rescue the minds of the most timid and foreboding from those agitations of the nervous system which greatly predispose the constitution to the

influence of contagious disease.³⁶

Religion and moral beliefs in part accounted for the cool manner in which the middle classes responded to the threat of cholera. Many achieved personal stability during the uncertainties of the epidemic and stayed to carry on their ordinary business or help with anti-cholera measures, because they were confident that God offered them eternal salvation if not total security in their temporal life. The experience of two Sheffield men bears this out. In early July 1832, John Holland, poet, journalist and newspaper editor, was sent from Sheffield to Newcastle to edit a new paper. He was clearly terrified by the cholera on the Tyne and worried by the epidemic which broke in Sheffield after he left, for his mother lived in one of the worst-affected areas.

> The tidings of mortality which every morning brought to my ears were most appalling. . .I felt a deep awe resting upon me during this reign of terror, and strove as well as I could to rest my mind upon that good and wise Being who has preserved me hitherto. . .³⁷

When James Montgomery, another newspaper editor and poet, decided to stay in Sheffield, he wrote to his friend, George Bennett, 'I find assurance in that book which contains the words of eternal life — "Thou wilt keep him in perfect peace, whose mind is stayed on thee, because he trusted in thee".'³⁸ The calming influence of religion had a social as well as a medical effect, for during the epidemic it gave many men the courage they needed to fulfil their social roles in the face of sudden death.

There was considerable evidence that God's purpose in sending cholera was being fulfilled and people were recalled to religion. To put the matter more sociologically, religious revival thrived in conditions of social instability and physical danger, as men needed to reassert their values and seek security in the promises and community of faith. Church attendance improved as the epidemic approached. At Sedgley, Girdlestone found more shops closing on Sunday and a decrease in bull-baiting. Marriages increased in the cholera quarter of the year. Cupid did not arrive with the miasma but the sickness and fear aroused by cholera roused the conscience of many who had long lived together unmarried and induced them to conform to the moral standards of the church.³⁹

The revival was greatest among the Methodists for they appealed to people of lower status who were most at risk during the epidemic and had a living tradition of recruiting large numbers by revival preaching. The revivals were in County Durham, along the Tyne, in the Black Country and in the declining lead-mining district of Chewton Mendip in Somerset. After the explosive outbreak at Gateshead in late 1831, the chapels were filled and 300 new members admitted. At Walbottle, a prayer meeting in a widow's house drew people from a riotous dance and began a revival which brought 60 probationers to the local congregation. A particularly impressive prayer meeting and the epidemic in nearby Newburn sparked off that sense of sin and loving redemption which was the basis of such revivals. The chapels of the Wednesbury circuit were full as cholera spread through Tipton, Dudley, Bilston and Sedgley,

> Meetings were held every evening of the week, and the chapel was filled: many groaned under a sense of their sin and guilt, sought mercy with cries and tears, and would hardly leave the chapel at a late hour.

The cholera revivals did not take place in the big towns and cities but in small mining communities affected by the disease. In these villages existing Methodist communities were in contact with those who ignored religion. Without the countless cross-pressures and counter-attractions which sophisticated even the poorest town-dweller, the village miner and his neighbours were more easily swept from the tensions of the epidemic to the emotion of revival.[40]

There was a traditional, quiet strand of Anglican thought which was less noisy than the evangelicals but certainly more effective. They were the Church and State men, orthodox, usually Tory in politics, certainly conservative in the wider meaning of that word. They reflected little on their religion. It was a matter of constitutional propriety rather than metaphysics. Religion was a civic affair, accepted for the stability and ceremony with which it provided society. On one hand, they feared the disruption caused by liberals and radicals who wanted to reform Parliament, emancipate Catholics, or worse still, reform the Church itself. On the other, they saw the dangerous 'enthusiasm' of the evangelicals, who would make religion a matter of personal contact between man and his God, without the necessary intervention of the state and the traditional structures of the Church. For the evangelical, the most important social relationship of all was that between God and man; the traditional Anglican paid more attention to the countless social relationships which maintained the eighteenth-century hierarchy of power with the bishops as part of the ruling class and the clergy as their aides. The Privy Council put the clergy in their traditional social role when they asked them to become members of the local boards of health along with other bearers of local authority. Henry Phillpotts, Bishop of Exeter, was criticised for neglecting this role by his archdeacon, George Barnes,

> Never was Exeter in such an emergency, never has there been such an awful visitation amongst us, and yet never was the Cathedral so deserted by Canons...The cry is, Where is the Bishop?...Are the Canons to receive their £700 a year merely to be present in their own routine of residence? Ought they not at such a crisis at least to be present to assist with their influence and advice, to encourage and support, to be free with their money, and to be ready to co-operate with the civil authorities?[41]

The Bishop and his canons were expected to stay and do their duty as part of the local ruling class, providing paternal care and leadership to the community in times of crisis, especially, as Barnes was painfully aware, because local radicals were eager to take the chance of attacking a Bishop who had voted against the Reform Bill.

The traditional Anglicans paid due respect to the part which Providence played in the epidemic but made little fuss about sin and causation. If there was any special sin it was radicalism,

> It [cholera] attacks those moral constitutions which have been weakened or undermined either by poverty of nutriment, or by too free use of those potent drugs and preparations which are distilled and rectified in the laboratory of modern liberalism.

Their God was an interventionist God, but in fact didn't intervene very often. Most plagues, conquests, revolutions, famines and wars, 'are within the ordinary powers of what man calls nature'. They may be produced by the undisturbed action of what man calls secondary causes. The day of miracles may, indeed, have ceased among us;...'But this I know — that, without baring his right arm, the Almighty can secretly so modify all elemental combination, or so direct the career of man's blind passions, that the result shall work together for the fulfilment of God's will.'[42] The orthodox Anglicans praised everything the government did as just and sensible, and advised everyone to be calm. Prayer was valued for its calming effect on the population as much as for its influence in placating an angry God. They waited for the government to issue official prayers and appoint national fast days and were mildly critical of those like Girdlestone, who ignored authority and appointed their own day.[43] Theirs was the mood which pervaded government, national and local board of health propaganda — 'an opportunity is presented to the charitable for the spontaneous performance of many Christian duties', the Oxford Board of Health had said before plunging into the practical details of a subscription, — it was a nod at the altar before getting on with day-to-day tasks of administration. It was a mood ideally suited to a ruling class seeking stability. This group went furthest in preserving the eighteenth-century, Cartesian division between religion and science. They did this by the simple expedient of the Tory throughout the ages — using the power they had and not asking too many unnecessary questions. Their position might be briefly stated, fear God, honour the King, keep quiet and don't ask questions.

Roman Catholic sources made little comment on the epidemic, but the views of Father Green of Birmingham must have been characteristic of the Catholic priesthood in the local parishes. In some ways his position was a pale reflection of the Broad Church Anglican. He had the same conservative respect for authority but took his lead from the Roman hierarchy rather than the bishops in the House of Lords when it came to prayers and fasting. His God shared many of the qualities of the avenging interventionist God of the Protestants. He advised his people to 'propitiate an offended God' with prayers and 'sentiments of contrition and penance'. Father Green could hardly accept the motivation which the evangelicals attributed to an angry God. If famine, disease and political disaster were divine punishment for sin, then British and Irish Catholics must be the worst of sinners. Cholera was not sent to punish sin but to test the faith and courage of those who were threatened by it. The Catholic priests were without the family ties of most Protestant ministers and clergy. Most lived in the Irish Catholic areas of the large industrial towns and acted as 'the good shepherd', continuing to visit their people during the epidemic. Father Green listed the many priests who risked their lives in the epidemic, and those Protestants, like Leigh of Sedgley, who had closed their churches and stopped visiting the sick. The Birmingham priest had nothing but contempt for this gesture to Board of Health regulations. St John has said that the hireling who was not the good Shepherd would fly from his sheep when the wolf came and this was just what had happened.[44]

The official day of fasting, prayer and humiliation on 21 March 1832 evoked the full range of religious responses to the cholera. The evangelicals greeted the day as government recognition of all their beliefs about the efficacy of prayer.[45] The bishops all preached in important places. Blomfield spoke optimistically in the Royal Chapel; 'When Thy judgments are in the earth, the inhabitants of the earth will learn righteousness' (Isaiah), and reminded his Royal audience that the rulers of society had neglected 'to increase the comforts and improve the moral character of the masses'.[46] Churches were full all over the country though opinion varied as to how far fear or genuine repentance was behind this. The poet Southey, vegetating in pacific Anglicanism, wrote from Keswick, 'The fast day produced a good effect here: profligate as this little town is, the church has never been better attended...'[47] The day was a communal expression of opposition to the disease. Administration and science had failed, so the nation reached back to more primitive and traditional means of expressing its feelings. Today a public enquiry would propitiate the need to 'do something' in the face of disaster, but when this was suggested in 1832, Poulett-Thompson rejected the idea. Society did not yet have enough confidence in its experts and scientists to allow them to perform the ritual dance of concern.

This fasting was not all it seemed. The *British Critic* admitted 'the appearance of salt fish and parsnips...is little more than a fragment of ancient custom'.[48] The Unitarians dismissed it as 'the tribute of political expediency to sectarian cant',

> We see not in our vision a puissant and devout nation kneeling in singleness of heart before its own undivided altar...There can be nothing like this in the harsh, vulgar, and discordant reality which is soon to be presented to our senses. The Fast Day will come, and people will leave off working, but nobody will abstain from eating, save those whom poverty compels to keep perennial fast. Even from them it may be presumed, charity will not withhold the soup which is distributed the more vigorously in the hope that it may help to keep the cholera from the neighbourhood. The theatres will close, the churches will be open, and the shops will manage their shutters so as to hit the happy medium. Amongst the higher classes a handsome dish of salt fish, at the head of a well spread table, by way of addition not substitution, will suffice to mark the day decorously.[49]

The working-class radical papers rocked with derision, contempt and a

Religion and Morals 149

rich invective which they had developed to a fine art. 'God', it seemed, was a ruling-class agent and hence to be ignored. Cobbett, Hetherington and the speakers at the National Union of the Working Classes meetings in Finsbury were all agreed, .

> Here's a precious piece of humbuggery! What a delectable treat it will be to peruse the prayer, composed for the occasion by our 'most Reverend', and Sinful, and Plundering Archbishops!!!
>
> 'A public day of fasting and humiliation!' What does this mean! the rich are not to eat meat, but to limit themselves to such food as "the earth and the waters under the earth" can accommodate them with (that is, every variety of fish − eggs − vegetables − fruit and wine, which wealth can procure and ingenuity render agreeable to the palate), while the poor, how are they to fast? − to do with less than they do as present, would be absolutely to starve. . .−no, no; to tell the poor to fast would indeed be superfluous.[50]

Few radicals could resist the opportunity which the fast day presented. Hetherington urged that 'The poor and destitute [should] assemble in the streets on the fast day and meet the saintly hypocrites by the thousand as they are going to church.' The members of the National Union marched around London, clashed with the police, several leaders were arrested and the rest sat down to dinners of roast beef subscribed for by the wealthier members. The First Salford Co-operative agreed with the medical men who thought that want of food was a cause of cholera, and invited all 'working classes' to a general feast. In Carlisle, the weavers adapted the ritual of friendly society and trades union to the occasion. They paraded the town with banners, fifes and drums. The banners were all relevant to the purpose of the day; cause of cholera, herring and three loaves; cure of cholera, roast beef and a loaf of bread; NO CANT. In the evening, they burnt Mr Perceval in effigy and a man mounted on a cross read a chapter from 'The Book of Weft', and concluded with a long prayer, 'the burthen of which was a call upon the Almighty to visit his wrath upon those who had been the oppressors of the people by keeping them from the bounties of his Providence.'[51] There was a note of sadness amongst all this abuse. The radicals made a few desperate attempts to appeal to their God over the heads of bishops and ruling classes who had stolen the Almighty from them,

> nor is it probable that our government would consider it at all likely

that an Almighty God could condescend to acknowledge, as worthy
of attention, the objects which itself, in its relative insignificance,
looks down upon with the most utter contempt'.[52]

In November, Hetherington had asked, 'What right have these practical
mockers and blasphemers to ask their Master for mercy, when they deny
it to all their own dependants'? The government's willingness to blame
the Almighty for disease and distress which was man-made, was regarded
by all the radicals as blasphemy. In the Painite tradition, they attacked
the Church, rejected the God of cholera as an agent of class oppression
without ever quite giving up hope of finding some 'Divine Being' of
infinite goodness to which they could appeal for justice.

The religious feelings aroused by the cholera provided Parliament
with a series of squalid little debates which took place against the
backdrop of the massive Reform Bill debates which occupied a tense
House night after night. The series was opened by Spencer Perceval, a
man of strong religious views, son of the Prime Minister who had been
assassinated in 1812. He told the Commons,

> He rose to address them in the name of the Lord Jesus Christ, the
> Saviour of the world, who was exalted King of Kings, and Lord of
> Lords. . .God, too, was present among them, and he would
> witness all that passed. . .he that rejected him [Mr. Perceval]
> rejected his God in whose name he appeared. . .

With the full range of evangelical arguments, he gained Althorp's 'tardy
consent' to the fast day. Althorp preferred his religion kept within
church doors as the mild assistant of government, but his attempts to
avoid the subject all failed. The debate over the Cholera Acts gave
Althorp similar trouble. One of the Surrey MPs wanted the preamble
amended to acknowledge that 'it hath pleased Almighty God' to visit
the kingdom with cholera and that preventative measures were being
taken with 'Divine Blessing'. The Bill went on its way without the
blessing of Providence, but when a similar amendment was suggested
for the Cholera Bill (Scotland) the following night it was accepted
without a murmur. Hume upset the evangelicals by calling the whole
thing 'cant, hypocrisy and humbug' and claimed that it was tough on the
Almighty to attribute special blame for cholera when He was responsible
for everything. Hunt didn't see why the Scots should monopolise
Providence, but in the Lords, the Bishop of London spoilt this fitting
inequality by firmly putting Providence into both preambles.[53]

Perceval was a member of Edward Irving's congregation in Regent Square. In late 1831, members of this congregation had been heard to speak with unknown tongues – as on the day of Pentecost. Members became increasingly fascinated by Irving's prophecy that the second coming of Christ was imminent and cholera would turn England into a charnel house in preparation for this event.[54] The night before the Fast he broke up the debate on the third reading of the Reform Bill demanding that the government pay more attention to the Divine purpose of cholera. Althorp failed to get the House adjourned. Some MPs trooped out in noisy disgust, others begged Perceval to sit down, evidently feeling some sympathy for a mind which was breaking under the tension between his powerful apocalyptic expectations of the second coming, and the secular unconcern with which his fellow MPs regarded the relationship of God and man. But the cholera had set fire to this explosive theological mixture and the thunder went on,

> I tell you this land will soon be desolate; a little time and ye shall howl one and all in the streets. I tell ye that pestilence which God is now holding in, will be let loose among ye and that the sword will follow...for be ye assured that the storm is coming, and he is nigh, who is at once your God, your Saviour and your judge.[55]

At one extreme cholera confirmed prophecies of the second advent, at the other it left men worrying about the burden on the rates, and how best to satisfy the etiquette of fast day.

The symbols which are a part of any religion's belief system are part of the cultural apparatus of symbols by which men transmit meaning to each other and perpetuate and develop their knowledge of the world about them. Sacred symbols give a comprehensive view of world order. Man cannot live in chaos. His religion and its symbols are his guide to reality when he predicts, makes judgements and takes action. They explain the events of life, and create, reinforce and explain feelings, moods, actions and morality needed to deal with these situations. Thus a society's use of religious symbols reflects their perception of physical and social reality.[56] The major symbol used to explain cholera was that of an all-powerful, sin-avenging, angry and terrible God. This uncompromising and awe-inspiring figure was decked out with all the elemental imagery of the Old Testament, with fire, with the noise of chariot wheels and rushing waters. The winter attack on Gateshead was likened to 'the lightening down of Jehovah's arm with the indignation of his anger, and with the flame of devouring fire; and he caused his glorious voice to be heard (Isaiah, ch.30, v.30).'[57]

Such a concept of God was meaningful to people who had little control over their lives. Most lacked all social and political independence. All faced high death rates and inescapable pain. Christ 'the adorable redeemer', the intermediary between man and his avenging God, had a minor role in confronting cholera. Religious and metaphysical beliefs are most valuable to men in times of stress. They turn to them in an attempt to gain control of a frightening situation. Christ the redeemer was the agent which gave men control in the face of cholera for he was 'the Prince of Life', 'the hope of life eternal', who emancipated his followers from the fear of death. The more human Christ of love and charity, the Christ of 'give all thou hast to the poor', was rarer in his appearances. Girdlestone preached from 'I was sick and ye visited me' but cholera gave little scope for the gentler parts of the Christian religion. The last major and potent symbol presented to the fearful public was that of mankind at prayer, humble, devout and repentant, a desperate ritual enactment of helplessness in a dangerous situation, but a ritual which ended with a claim on greater powers to assert control.

Swirling around these great concepts of God, Christ and prayer was a selection of that host of minor symbols relished by Protestant Britain, the stories of the Old and New Testaments. The 'destroying angel' appeared in many dissertations on cholera, and the actions of this aide of Almighty God were illustrated with a varied collection of pestilence texts from the Old Testament. 'The leader of the host was employed in the land of Egypt', said the *Congregational Magazine;* another visited the camp in the wilderness, and destroyed 'the crown of pride, the drunkards of Ephraim'; fornication, the delight in war and neglect of the Lord were all causes of pestilence. The Reformed Presbyterians began their warnings with the tale of Sodom and Gommorrah, then delivered a volley of pestilence texts with breathtaking speed and economy of words,

> . . ., Lev.xxvi.25, When you are gathered together within your cities. I will send the pestilence among you, He is declared to smite with it (Num.xiv.12), cause it to cleave to a people (Duet.xxviii.21) and to give over their life to its power (Ps.lxxviii 50). . .[58]

The link between God's might and cholera and sin was hammered home in text after text. But the books of the Bible provided countless assurances that such afflictions were intended to recall men to God and that prayer would be answered. The story of Nineveh was referred to time and again. When threatened with destruction by the Lord for various misdeeds, the people of Nineveh declared a fast and put on sack cloth,

> Jonah, Ch. 3, v.10. And God saw their works, that they turned from their evil way; and God repented of the evil, that He had said He would do unto them; and He did it not.

Everyone from Wesleyans to Presbyterians who read this text felt it was 'an instructive instance'. The *Christian Observer* was sure that God heard their prayers and 'commanded that our British Nineveh should not be destroyed'.[59] There were many, especially among the evangelicals, who saw the British nation as the spiritual inheritors of Israel as God's people. These minor symbols, the texts and Bible stories all played a supportive role, lending the authority of the Bible to the parts assigned to Almighty God, Christ and prayer in the explanation and response to cholera.

The belief structure concerning God and cholera may be related to two other social factors if each church or denomination is identified with the social status of its leadership and the access which that leadership had to constitutional power. Each group's belief in the extent of God's intervention in the affairs of man and cholera was related to the leadership's share of constitutional power. The two groups which felt themselves excluded from power both rejected the idea of God's direct intervention for the punishment of sin. The Unitarians and the working-class radicals were both agreed on this, although they were of very different levels of social status. The Unitarians were members of the middle-class urban élite, excluded from power because they rejected the Trinity. The increasing access to power which they had gained in the few years before 1832 would not have altered attitudes to science and society which had been formed by eighteenth-century traditions. The working-class radical leaders mostly came from the craft, skilled artisan margins of the middle and working classes, and were watching a political scene in which Whig reformers and Tory anti-reformers both seemed to be ignoring the claims of their working-class followers.

Those who had power accepted that God had a direct part in the cholera. The ruling classes of England and Scotland had authority and responsibility for taking immediate decisions about the welfare and security of the population of Britain. They could not afford the luxury of the out-groups who rejected God-based explanations of cholera. The men in government wanted immediate, authoritative and convincing explanations of what was happening, so they could take the necessary decisions with confidence. At the same time, they had a limited amount of medical and scientific knowledge and few of the resources to make use of this knowledge. They needed to protect their own authority from individual and group challenge from those of lower status, so that God's part in the cholera and the anti-cholera campaign was limited. His Almighty authority was exercised through the ruling classes. There were other groups who had less share of constitutional power. The Anglican evangelicals were vicars and curates rather than bishops. The Congregationalists and Wesleyans were more likely to be members of parish vestries than Members of Parliament. They had authority and responsibility but scant resources. They needed the intervention of God to give them confidence, but accepted this intervention to a far greater degree than their social superiors because they had less power themselves. The Roman Catholics fit uneasily into this pattern. They had no direct constitutional power. The Father Greens of the Roman Church were both poor and without the vote, yet they had great authority over their own people, and accepted the responsibility that went with this. Their own authority led them to a respect for all social authority and for the *status quo*, hence their God of cholera was an all-powerful, purposeful and interventionist God, but without the detailed intervention of the evangelical God who sat on the thunder-cloud picking his victims with such individual care. Catholic power might have been a pale shadow of the Anglican Church but their assumptions about social authority and the part played by God in the exercise of this authority were much the same.

The second social dimension of the relationship between God and cholera showed that the sins which were specified as the objects of God's wrath were described with more exactness as the social status of the leadership fell. Now the imperatives of religion tend to be functional. This does not mean that a man will choose his religious beliefs with a careful eye to his own advantage. It means that an individual or group will be attracted by and retain a series of religious beliefs which seem relevant to the upbringing, life style, responsibilities and worries of the individual or group concerned. Religious beliefs tend to maintain the structure and stability of society as seen from the point of view of the individual or group. Thus, sin is that action which tends to disrupt social stability and confidence. Each part of society will again have different perspectives for choosing those actions which seem most dangerous to its own security. Thus those at the top of the social scale can afford to be vague about sin. For their own stability the élite need little more than the loyalty of their subjects, which translated into religious terms meant faith and worship in accordance with the dictates of the bishops and elders. The middle-class sects, like the Congregationalists, had to be a little more exacting. Sin for them was the neglect of hard work, for many of them were manufacturers and traders whose prosperity depended on qualities of work and diligence. Other groups like the Methodists, Reformed Presbyterians, even the working-class radicals, had to be more specific. They lived on the borderline of the middle and working classes. They lived with high standards of respectability and independence but scant resources. Personal faults like drink, gambling, or even misfortunes outside their control like sickness or a fall in wages and employment could make all the difference between an orderly and comfortable life and disaster and poverty. Hence their sins were detailed specific personal faults like drinking, dog-baiting, and neglect of chapel; usually these sins involved some loss of self-control, for rigid self-control was essential for maintaining personal independence when the margin between order and disaster was so narrow. The Reformed Presbyterian added the threats of Popery to their own list of disasters for they were Lowland and Ulster Scots who felt their security threatened by the immigration of Irish Catholics into the growing industrial areas of Glasgow and Belfast. The 'countenancing of idolatry' had a special personal meaning to the readers of *The Covenanter*, though it was only a mildly irritating challenge to authority for the readers of the *British Critic*. The working-class radical had his own perspective. The tax-eating aristocratic sinecurist and the reactionary bishops and the poverty of their followers threatened the order and security of their lives quite as much as cholera could do.

The relationship between religious and social factors was by no means an exact one. Being evangelical still had more influence on a man's interventionist views than his social status and authority, but the relationship was close enough to suggest that status and power did have some influence on a debate which essentially was still between religious groups.

Notes

1. Keith Thomas, *Religion and the Decline of Magic*, London, 1971;
   E. Evans-Pritchard, *Nuer Religion*, London, 1956.
2. Emile Durkheim, *The Elementary Forms of Religious Life*, London, 1915;
   M. Weber, 'Major Features of World Religions', first published 1915, reprinted

in *Sociology of Religion,* Roland Robertson (ed.), London, 1969;
N. Abercrombie *et al.,* 'Superstition and Religion; the God of the Gaps' in *A Sociological Yearbook of Religion in Britain,* no.3, David Martin and Michael Hill (eds.), pp.93-129.
3. Elie Halévy, *England in 1815,* London, 1924, pp.387-484; Owen Chadwick, *The Victorian Church,* 2 vols., London, 1966; W.R. Ward, *Religion and Society in England, 1790-1850,* London, 1972; H.J. Perkin, *The Origins of Modern English Society,* London, 1969, pp.196-207; J.H.S. Burleigh, *A Church History of Scotland,* Oxford, 1960.
4. J.D. Bernal, *Science in History,* 3 vols., 1954, vol.2, pp.445-7; Thomas Paine, *The Age of Reason,* London, 1937, introduction by Chapman Cohen (originally published 1794); (William Hone), *The Political House that Jack Built,* London, 1819 and *The Political Showman at Home,* London, 1821; (Richard Carlile), *The order for the administration of loaves and fishes, or the communion of corruptions host. . .,* London, 1820, pp.140 and 219-89; G.J. Holyoake, *Sixty Years of an Agitator's Life,* 2 vols., London, 1892, vol.II, p.292, and *The Life and Character of Richard Carlile,* London, 1853, p.24.
5. T.H. Huxley, *Science and the Christian Tradition,* London, 1894, vol.10 of *Collected Essays,* preface and pp.32-7; Leonard Huxley, *Life and Letters of Thomas Henry Huxley,* 3 vols., London 1903, vol.1, pp.313-18; C.G. Gillespie, *Genesis and Geology,* Harvard, 1951; Walter Cannon, 'The problem of miracles in the 1830's', *Victorian Studies,* vol.4, 1960, p.228.
6. F.K. Brown, *Fathers of the Victorians,* Cambridge, 1961; Owen Chadwick, *The Victorian Church;* W.R. Ward, *Religion and Society.*
7. *Wesleyan Methodist Magazine,* vol.12, 3rd series, p.21. Hereafter referred to as *W.M.M.*
8. *Congregational Magazine,* vol.15, 1832, p.158; *Missionary Magazine,* 1832, pp.373 and 412; *W.M.M.,* vol.55, 1832, pp.258 and 714.
9. *Christian Observer,* vol.32, 1832, p.124.
10. *The Evangelical Magazine and Missionary Chronicle,* new series, vol.10, 1832, p.22.
11. *Christian Observer,* vol.32, 1832, p.125.
12. *W.M.M.,* 3rd series, vol.11, 1832, pp.260-1 and 273; *The Covenanter,* vol.2, Belfast and Glasgow, 1832, p.268.
13. *Christian Observer,* vol.34, 1834, p.12.
14. *Congregational Magazine,* vol.15, 1832, p.157.
15. *W.M.M.,* vol.11, 3rd series, 1832, pp.204-5.
16. These reflections are based on B.H. Harrison, *Drink and the Victorians,* London, 1971.
17. *Cholera Gazette,* no.2, 28 January 1832; Henry Gaulter, *Malignant Cholera in Manchester,* p.37.
18. *Directions for the Prevention and Cure of Cholera Morbus as suggested by the Board of Health President, Sir Henry Halford,* published by H.M. Privy Council, London, 1831; *Directions to Plain People for their Conduct during the Cholera,* London, 1831; John Goss, *Practical Remarks on the Disease called Cholera which now exists on the continent of Europe,* London, 1831; T.W. Chevalier, *On Asiatic Cholera,* London, 1831; *E.M.S.J.,* vol.37, p.219, the handbills in the Radcliffe Infirmary collection in Oxford and many other similar titles and sources; *Fraser's Magazine,* vol.4, 1831, p.625; *Monthly Review,* vol.3, 1831, p.459; *Poor Man's Guardian,* 7 January 1832; *Poor Man's Advocate,* 18 August 1832.
19. *Evangelical Magazine,* vol.9, 1831, p.572; *Christian Observer,* vol.34, 1834, pp.2-3; *W.M.M.,* vol.55, 1832, p.203; *The Covenanter,* vol.2, Belfast and Glasgow, 1832, p.269; *The Congregational Magazine,* vol.15, 1832.

Religion and Morals 157

20. *Edinburgh Courant*, 6 September 1832; John Snow, *On the mode of communication of Cholera*, London, 1855, 2nd edition, p.43.
21. George Watt, 'On the origin and spread of malignant cholera in Glasgow and its neighbourhood', *Glasgow Medical Journal*, vol.5, 1832, p.388.
22. R. Pollitzer, *Cholera*, p.291; My thanks to Dr. A.G. Leitch, Department of Medicine, Edinburgh University, for his help with this section.
23. *C.O.*, vol.32, 1832, p.125; *W.M.M.*, vol.2, 3rd series, 1832, p.382.
24. *C.O.*, vol.32, 1832, p.627; *W.M.M.*, vol.2, 3rd series, 1832, p.382.
25. *Congregational Magazine*, vol.15, 1832, p.72.
26. E. Durkheim, *The Elementary Forms of Religious Life*, London, 1915, p.429.
27. *C.O.*, vol.34, 1834, pp.1-16; *W.M.M.*, 1832, p.275; *The Covenanter*, vol.2, Belfast and Glasgow, 1832, p.265.
28. *W.M.M.*, 3rd series, vol.2, 1832, p.259 and vol.10, 1831, p.791; *The Covenanter*, vol.2, Belfast and Glasgow, 1832.
29. *C.O.*, vol.34, 1834, p.12.
30. *Congregational Magazine*, vol.15, March 1832.
31. *C.O.*, vol.32, 1832; *Evangelical Magazine*, vol.9, 1831, p.531; *Presbyterian Magazine*, vol.1, Edinburgh, 1832.
32. *Missionary Register*, 1832, p.329, printing the 28th Annual Report of the British and Foreign Bible Society; *C.O.*, vol.34, 1834, p.7.
33. *The Monthly Repository*, vol.4, new series, 1830, p.151 and vol.6, new series, 1832, pp.10, 47 and 150-1.
34. *W.M.M.*, 1832, p.259 and 1833, p.21.
35. Thomas Jackson, *The Life of the Rev. Robert Newton, D.D.*, London, 1855, p.125.
36. *Evangelical Magazine*, vol.9, 1831, p.533; and vol.10, 1832, p.108.
37. William Hudson, *The Life of John Holland of Sheffield Park*, London, 1874, p.169.
38. John Holland and James Everett, *Memoirs of James Montgomery*, 7 vols., London, 1856, vol.5, p.54, letter dated 10 August 1832.
39. *C.O.*, vol.33, 1833, pp.445-511.
40. *W.M.M.*, 1832, pp.216-17, 275, 449-50, 662 and 748; J.W. Gough, *Mines of Mendip*, Newton Abbott, 1867, pp.170-231.
41. G.C.B. Davies, *Henry Phillpotts, Bishop of Exeter, 1778-1869*, London, 1954, pp.140-4; Rev. Reginald N. Shutte, *The Life, times and writing of the Rt. Rev. Henry Phillpotts, Lord Bishop of Exeter*, London, 1863, pp.406-15.
42. *The British Critic*, vol.11, 1832, pp.376 and 384.
43. *The British Magazine*, 1832, p.387.
44. *The Catholic Magazine and Review*, vol.4, Birmingham, 1833, pp.65-89.
45. *Christian Observer*, vol.32, 1832, pp.124-5; *W.M.M.*, 1832, p.257.
46. Rev. George Edward Biber, *Bishop Blomfield and his times*, London, 1857, pp.129-34.
47. John Warter Wood, *Selections from the letters of Robert Southey*, 4 vols., London, 1856, vol.4, p.269.
48. *The British Critic*, vol.11, 1832, pp.377-9.
49. *The Monthly Repository*, new series, vol.6, 1832, p.145; George Harris, *Public Fasts Irrational...*, Glasgow, March 1832.
50. *Poor Man's Guardian*, 12 November 1832; *Cobbett's Political Register*, 10 December 1831.
51. *Poor Man's Guardian*, 11 February and 31 March 1832; P. Hollis, *The Pauper Press*, Oxford, 1970, p.45.
52. *Poor Man's Guardian*, 11 February 1832.
53. *Hansard's Parliamentary Debates*, 3rd series, vol.10, 16 February 1832.
54. E. Miller, *History of Irvingism*, 2 vols., London, 1878; Mrs Oliphant, *Life*

of *Edward Irving*, 2 vols., London, 1862.
55. *Hansard's Parliamentary Debates*, 3rd series, vol.11, 20 March 1832.
56. Clifford Geertz, 'Religion as a cultural system' in M. Banton (ed.), *Anthropological Approaches to Religion*, London, 1966, pp.1-44.
57. *W.M.M.*, 1832, p.275.
58. *The Covenanter*, vol.1, Belfast and Glasgow, 1832, pp.263-8.
59. *Christian Observer*, vol.33, 1833, p.445.

8 MEDICINE AND SCIENCE

The only real hope of stopping cholera lay with the medical profession. There were two basic problems, treating patients who caught cholera, and preventing the disease spreading to others.

(i) The Doctors

The medical profession was ill-equipped socially and technically to deal with either of these problems. It was fragmented and suffering the tensions and jealousies of change from an ancient art to a science-based profession.

In the eighteenth century, the medical profession had crystallised into three formal ranks. The physician, supposed only to prescribe medicine, was the aristocrat of the profession. He was a member of the Royal College, which was dominated by the Fellows, all graduates of Oxford or Cambridge. They all had a gentleman's education, which included little medical content. But as medicine could do little for the patient in the eighteenth century, this was not a great omission. The surgeon was the tradesman of medicine. He worked with his hands and was supposed to call the physician if any prescribing was to be done. The Surgeon's Company was formed in 1745, gained a Royal Charter in 1800, and was dominated by the men who held posts in the growing number of London hospitals. The apothecaries were the servant class of medicine; officially they had to wait for the orders of a physician before prescribing medicine. Their status had recently been enhanced by the Apothecaries Act of 1815, which gave them monopoly rights over the examination and granting of qualifications in England. Two developments were confusing this carefully ordered pattern of a stratified profession. Most apothecaries were working as general practitioners (the word was first used in 1815). They prescribed drugs as well as mixing and selling them. Many surgeons and physicians who did not have lucrative posts in London hospitals or did not command the high incomes of wealthy fee-paying practices were also in general practice. In addition, a large number of Scots medical graduates came south, and in the north of England they dominated general practice. The best of them came from Edinburgh and Glasgow which, since the middle of the eighteenth century, had provided a science-based medical education superior to anything in England, but the Scots doctors included graduates of St Andrews and Aberdeen who might have purchased their degrees for £24.8s.11d., a course open to those who had failed exams elsewhere. In this confusion the different sections of the profession fought for power in a way which hindered co-operation against cholera and gained little public confidence.[1]

The body-snatching riots and the cholera riots were only one aspect of mounting public distrust of the medical men. Many readers of the unstamped Press in the 1830s distrusted the profession as charlatans. Hetherington quoted the stewardess of a London Friendly Society, 'I am no friend of the doctors. They are like lawyers, who will give an opinion on the side which pays them best.' Doctors, she thought, 'have been sent upon earth to scourge the sons and daughters of men with cholera and other fatal diseases'.[2] The radical journalists of the middle classes still mocked the doctor as an ignorant man unable to cure but willing to take fees and legacies from his patients.[3]

This crisis in the relationship between doctors and public arose from two changes in the doctor's work situation. There was a rising demand for medical attention among the middle classes as their increasing wealth enabled them to pay higher fees. At the same time, the profession was taking a more scientific interest in its subject matter. By the 1820s, following up John Hunter's work, doctors had a full knowledge of all parts of the body which could be studied without the aid of a microscope. In the early 1800s an increasing number of professional journals began to appear with details of case histories, autopsies, epidemic surveys, surgical techniques and medical theories. This scientific attitude filtered through to a wider public in newspapers and periodical reports. The public began to expect the doctor to be more than adviser and comforter and to use his science to prevent and cure. The doctor could do little to satisfy the expectations created by his increase in scientific knowledge for this was not matched by any substantial advance in therapy until the introduction of antiseptic techniques in the 1870s and 1880s. Before then, the only real opportunities for reducing sickness and death rates lay with public health measures which had a low prestige with the profession.

Cholera deepened this crisis in relationships between doctors and people. 'Who shall decide when doctors disagree,' asked Doherty, as he considered with dismay their failures and their disputes over the nature, treatment and even the identity of cholera. With its usual informed drawing-room concern the *New Monthly Review* greeted the doctor's efforts with a discreet screech of contempt, 'Of all classes that have ever distinguished themselves for absurdity, none have ever exceeded the doctors. The history of medicine is a history of folly and quackery...'[4] Those who visited the north-east of England in late 1831 reported an increasing loss of confidence among the people there, as the doctors' advice grew more confused and contradictory. The radicals continued to accuse the doctors of falsehood, exaggeration, jobbery and distortion for political purposes. They reported with glee the more absurd mistakes. The surgeon in Glasgow who confused pregnancy pains with the onset of cholera was an especial favourite.[5] *Carpenter's* admitted that the misdeeds of the 'venial' had been countered by 'the manly and independent exertions of the better part of the profession', indicating that they did recognise the professional standards being pressed by men like Charles Hastings, leader of the Provincial Medical and Surgical Association and radicals like Thomas Wakeley in the *Lancet*. Religious commentators were equally scornful of the confusion and failure of the profession in the face of cholera.

> The leeches it is well known, are evermore an irritable race; and no-one can be surprised that a new medical problem should set their polemical propensities in immediate and violent action.[6]

The confusion and failure provided them with more proof of the power of God, and was a reason for the widespread acceptance of religious comfort and explanation during the epidemic. If the interventionist God was a God of the Gaps, then medical science and therapy left many gaps.

Any effective enquiry into the nature and causes of cholera was hampered by the absence of any research community in medicine. Such medical research as was done was carried out by the consultants in the London and provincial hospitals and by general practitioners, though, as Dodd in Houghton-le-Spring complained during 1832, they had little time for such activities. There was no social group which specialised in research. This situation, in which research and practice were combined, led to a great exchange of information on symptoms and treatments for all diseases, and to the increase in anatomical knowledge. Knowledge was accumulated about many of the common fevers and their relationship to locality, but for cholera there was no motive for sustained and intensive research. All the major hospitals excluded infectious diseases and amongst them cholera, so that the consultant surgeon and physician had little occasion to study cholera in the wards, and the ambitious young practitioner with his eye on being elected to a hospital post would see no link between publication on cholera – hospital post – reputation and rich fee-paying patients.

The GP, be he physician, surgeon or apothecary by official title, was no better placed. He might publish a rapid survey of existing knowledge with a few speculations and any case histories that came to his notice from Indian experience or a quick tour of north-east England and Scotland during the winter of 1831-2. By such means he could gain notice as the man who knew about cholera during the few months in which the fee-paying middle class and the surgeon hiring poor law overseers were worried and frightened by cholera. Once the epidemic had left, interest was retained only by those few men for whom natural curiosity, or a political interest in sanitary reform, provided a motive for writing up their notes and reflections on the epidemic. The likely relationship of publication and career success encouraged sporadic interest rather than sustained enquiry into cholera.

In two years of hectic debate and activity the doctors pulled together the full organisational, scientific and therapeutic resources of their calling and publicly failed to make any impression on the disease. This failure had its heroic moments. The *Edinburgh Evening Courant* asked if all the abuse was a 'fit manifestation of gratitude to men who, at hazard of their lives, are grappling with a distemper that is diffusing gloom and apprehension throughout the country'.[7] The task of the cholera medical man was demanding and exhausting. In December 1831 Daun had to stop work because of exhaustion. When Alison went from Edinburgh to Dumfries to help with the explosive outbreak there, his sense of anxiety grew with every call he made. He received continual requests to hurry along nearly deserted streets. On one occasion, making a second visit, he passed the hearse carrying away the body of his patient. After a few days, 'want of natural repose and perpetual anxiety, destroyed all desire for food'. He dosed himself with a 'suitable medicine' and 'sank into a delightful sleep' which lasted fifteen hours, and awoke fit for work. If anything, local medical men were in an even more unenviable position, for after cholera passed they had to live with any unpopularity they incurred. J. Barles, surgeon in Airdrie, admitted to the Central Board that because of the general feeling of hostility, no doctors 'who wish to stand well with the public' would recommend the measures needed to deal with cholera.[8] Despite the long hours they worked and the risks they took, the dominant impression the doctors left on the public mind was of squabbling, self-interest and failure.

(ii) Treatments

The vast literature of the epidemic offered a bewildering variety of

treatments. But each had its rationale, some in tradition, others in old
and new systems of science, whilst experience produced new empirically
tested treatments.

In the early months of the epidemic the traditional tactic of bleeding
the patient was basic to most courses of treatment. It was especially
popular amongst doctors with Indian experience. Bleeding had initially
been based upon the great system of humoral pathology which had
developed with various sophistications from the Middle Ages. This
system attributed all disease to an imbalance or impurity in the body
fluids. Treatment consisted of the removal of the offending fluids by
bleeding, purging and sweating.[9] It was characteristic of most of the
modes of treatment described here that they could be derived from
several of the available scientific theories. Thus the Edinburgh surgeon,
George Hamilton Bell, late residency surgeon in Tanjore, based his
recommendation on his observations and understanding of the pathology
of the disease. He observed that the circulation was impaired, and felt
the mechanical effect of bleeding was to restore the circulation, by
relieving the weakened system 'gorged' with blood. Bleeding was a
treatment which rapidly came in for criticism. Like the purgatives
which so often accompanied it, bleeding did nothing for the inflamed
bowels, wrote a London doctor to the *Lancet*.[10] Increasing numbers of
writers suggested that bleeding should only be used in the early stages
of cholera; then that it should never be used in cases of true cholera. The
theorists were all beaten by the harsh practical fact that as cholera
advanced in the bodies of its victims the savage dehydration meant that
very little was left to bleed, and several observers noted the black tarry
blood that was obtained in attempts to apply the traditional remedy.
Ainslie noticed that many abandoned the treatment. Experience of
cholera, he said, 'has shattered the faith of many believers'.[11]

Despite the violent purging of cholera itself, many courses of
treatment involved the use of laxatives to drive the poison from the
patients' bodies. At Leeds Robert Baker prescribed a castor oil
emulsion, and anticipated further purging then the restoration of natural
secretions.[12] Other doctors rejected this as being too violent and used
calomel which they felt was milder in its action. The purgatives could
be related to a different system. Dodd wrote from Houghton-le-Spring,
'I like others pursued the stimulating plan.'[13] Dodd advised castor oil,
magnesia and rhubarb – all these were standard items of the nineteenth-
century doctor's *materia medica*, with which he met the day-to-day
problems of stomach and bowels amidst the inadequate starchy food
and the contaminated water of urban and rural populations alike. The

stimulating system referred to another of the eighteenth-century systems of pathology. These monistic systems attributed all illness to one underlying state of the body, and hence looked for one basic system of treatment. In the tension pathology which Dodd had followed, illness was caused by the tone of the vascular or nervous systems — they might be overstimulated or depressed. If they were, counter-action had to be taken. Most observers agreed that cholera depressed the system. Both pulse and temperature could fall rapidly. Hence they countered this by stimulating the system. To the laxative they added a little brandy and occasionally small doses of opium. To counter the cold of the patient's skin, they applied heat in various ways. Hot bricks, linseed, mustard and bran poultice, a cataplasm of hayseeds and warm sand or salt were several of the methods used. Most practitioners rejected the simple hot bath of water as too exhausting for the patient. From this followed the hot air bath, a characteristic bit of cholera equipment. The one devised by Hamilton Bell was adopted by the Edinburgh Board of Health. A semi-cylindrical frame of open wicker work was placed over the patient's body and under the bedclothes. At the foot of the bed was an open copper tube, which bent over and presented a wide mouth over a large spirit flame. For six pennyworth of alcohol per hour the patient could be kept at a temperature of $120°$-$160°$F. This was clearly an expensive form of treatment only available for wealthy medical men and the better-equipped hospitals.

Many doctors followed the symptoms of the disease and attempted to combat each one as it arose. In the early days William Anderson, a surgeon, writing of the Bengal epidemic had said,

> In the treatment of cholera, our exertions must be turned to combat its influence by such remedies as are known to produce a contrary effect. In the present state of our knowledge all we can do is combat the symptoms.

The seventeenth-century physician, Sydenham, had laid the foundations of the English tradition of studying and classifying diseases according to their various symptoms. Many, like Anderson, used opium, the 'sheet anchor' of Sydenham's system, to combat the vomiting, purging and spasms produced by cholera.[14] Others used laudanum, a derivative of opium. Many of the other treatments fitted into this plan. Heat was used to combat the coldness of the skin, and various stimulants like brandy were used in the collapse stage. Some used violent emetics of mustard to clear the stomach of its contents. Others used enemas of tobacco to counter the poisons of the stomach.

Another group of medical men called the Broussian or pathological school traced the symptoms to their source in the organs of the body. This derived from the rational-empirical method of the *Ideologues* developed in the Paris hospitals after 1800. They broke down sickness into specific diseases, and followed Margagni's belief that diseases could be identified by the damage done to the organs of the body.[15] Because the dehydration of cholera did widespread damage to all parts of the body it was hard to be sure that cholera was indeed an infection of the bowels. Those who found it so did counter its effect with opium and brandy, with lime and water or with peppermint and ether. Others like Bell looked to the circulation and nervous system and attempted to revive them. This analytical approach led the men of 1832 the nearest they came to modern treatment in the work of O'Shaughnessy and Latta which relied on a saline infusion into the veins.

Most doctors used a combination of these treatments. The medical journals gave full accounts of their experience, but, as the *Edinburgh Medical and Surgical Journal* warned, no treatment from Moscow to Sunderland had made any impact on death rates. The medical profession was baffled by cholera. They tried the full contents of the medical chest with little result. Although it was natural for each man to try his existing treatments first, it was remarkable how adaptable and how ready to change most doctors were. The willingness to experiment in the heat of battle was one indicator of the shock impact which cholera had. *Tait's,* with the perception of an amateur, noted that the disease was always less virulent at the end than at the beginning of an epidemic and explained,

> Medical men who at first found all their drugs unavailing, have attributed to their last experimental medicines, cures which would have taken place although nothing had been administered.[16]

Thus a run of successes associated with a particular course of treatment would induce one doctor to place his faith in that system whilst the same methods would bring only death for another who would write to discredit the first. This experimentation brought into favour some novel treatments derived from the new sciences of pneumatic chemistry and electricity. Patients were given oxygen and wired up to galvanic batteries in an attempt to revive them. The only real agreement which the profession reached was that cholera should be treated early, preferably in the stage of preliminary diarrhoea. This added new

complications to any effective evaluation of cholera treatments for
many cases of quite ordinary diarrhoea were successfully treated as
potential cholera. To those who held a monistic theory of pathology,
the reasoning was quite simple, cholera had the same underlying cause
as other diseases, so that diarrhoea coming from the same cause might
develop into cholera and thus the preliminary symptoms needed to be
cut off before they developed. The posters and handbills all urged those
who suspected they might have cholera to come for early treatment.

The total picture of counter-measures and treatments was one of
irrational ignorance searching in a random way for effective action,
but each choice of drug, each choice of action can be understood in
the light of a complex of medical tradition, scientific method,
experience and principles of association, both primitive and philosophical.

(iii) Thomas Latta of Leith

The most effective life-saving treatment devised by the twentieth
century has been the injection of saline fluid into the veins of the
cholera patient. This counters the drastic dehydration caused by the
vibrio. This treatment was first proposed in 1832 by Dr Thomas Latta
of Leith. It was a reasoned deduction from careful scientific research.
It was published and discussed in the medical journals but never gained
widespread acceptance. The reasons for this lay in the limited resources
and techniques, in the limited scientific understanding and in the social
structure of authority and prestige in the medical profession.

In December 1831, Dr W.B. O'Shaughnessy published in the *Lancet*
the preliminary results of research he had carried out in Newcastle on
the blood of cholera victims. His analysis — made possible by the recent
advance and interest in analytical chemistry — showed that the blood of
cholera victims was seriously deficient in water and certain salts. His
report on 'The Chemical Pathology of Malignant Cholera' was received
by the Central Board of Health in December and under their authority
given further publicity in the medical journals.[17] This research was
followed up by Latta. The Leith doctor read the initial letter in the
Lancet and decided to restore the lost fluid and salts. He tried
administering his mixture orally and anally. Both failed, so he injected
the fluid into the veins with successful results. He reported that three
of his first five trial patients had lived. The *Lancet* welcomed the new
treatment, saying that it had saved lives. Others were not so sure. The
London Medical Gazette noted sourly that Latta's examples were the
only cases in which the saline method had achieved cures.[18]
Correspondents of both journals soon arrived with evidence that cast

doubt on Latta's methods and reasoning.

There were several reasons why a treatment so valuable in this century should have been largely ignored in 1832. The saline treatment fitted into none of the dominant medical traditions. Moreover, its originator was a man with little authority or prestige in the medical world he was trying to influence. Robert Lewins of 6 Quality Street, Leith, another doctor and close friend of Latta's, explained the circumstances to the Central Board of Health.

> The extra-ordinary practice alluded to and recommended in my former communication, has met with great I had almost said illiberal if not malignant opposition in Leith and Edinburgh. Latta is a worthy but rather obscure man — certain worthies attempted to frighten or bully him that he might not persist in his practice.

The social situation in which Latta found himself was an awkward one. His treatment was a deduction from the relatively new tradition of chemical pathology. Once he had made his breakthrough in therapy he was faced with the opposition of the defenders of the existing competing schools of thought. These defenders were powerful, experienced and prestigious men, leaders of the profession in Edinburgh. For a local doctor to challenge the opinion of leading physicians, surgeons and professors when the lives of his patients were at stake must have been a difficult and worrying task; but to gain from them an authoritative and fair assessment of the new treatment and space in the journals which those leaders controlled was well nigh impossible. Lewins continued the story of events as Latta prepared a paper for publication,

> the Edinburgh Board of Health, I mean the medical part of them, have behaved ill in this matter — I communicated the particulars of the first cases to Christison, Alison, Hamilton Bell and James Gregory, the two latter are the secretaries, about a week ago, but they have done nothing in the matter...
>
> Gregory, who is a tolerably acute man, but disagreeably dogmatic seemed at once to settle the matter in his own mind — that the practice referred to was inconsistent with physiological principles — that it was dangerous...

Gregory recommended that the Edinburgh Board should not use the saline treatment.

Lewins claimed that, if Latta's view had been listened to,

'tis probable that the injecting of the veins would have been practised sooner and many lives saved — And those men who stood in the way of scientific investigation at the period I refer to, in February and who, even now, refuse to try, or to recommend — aye or even to go and see the effects of a remedy capable of producing the wonderful effect in cholera that I have mentioned.

Lewins blamed the leading Edinburgh men, especially Dr Christison, for using their power to curb the development and publicity of Latta's work,

> he [Christison] had laid himself open to many animadversions — and he shall get it if I shall publish which I am resolved to do — I shall not spare him and his co-adjutors whose principal preliminary labours for which they take so much credit seem to have consisted in furnishing two or three hospitals with brooms, besoms, urinals and water pots, and in making matter for an extra number of the Edinburgh Journal which is now, I believe, Christison's private property exclusively.[19]

The clash between the two traditions of medicine was a tense one. At first all the points went to the prestige and power of the established authorities, but by the end of May, Lewins and Latta had persuaded the doctor at one of the Edinburgh cholera hospitals to try the treatment and Dr Graham, Professor of Botany, Christison and Alison witnessed the operation at the Drummond Street hospital where they were astonished at the rate of recovery and, Lewins claimed, all became converts.

The resistance of the Edinburgh doctors and the slow investigation and adoption of Latta's method was not surprising if his work was considered from the point of view of men who had been educated and worked all their lives in the traditions of the old pathologies. The type of response which the thoughtful and well-educated medical man might have been expected to make to Latta's ideas was set out by Dr James McCabe of Cheltenham in a letter to the Central Board,

> If we adopt in our explanation, the humoral pathology and suppose the cause of these discharges (of water and salts) to be the state or condition of the blood itself, we must also adopt the language of the old physiologists and refer to an acrimony of the blood and humours. What this acrimony can be unless it be an excess of

saline particles in the blood it is difficult to imagine. . .it is evident
that the saline injections would be a pathological contradiction.[20]

In other words, McCabe accepted all the evidence of the chemical
analysis but believed that if the body was getting rid of so much salt
and water it must be because there was an excess of this material in the
body, and to pump in more saline fluid was to confuse cause with effect
and quite possibly make the basic condition of the body worse. This
analysis cannot be contradicted on its own terms. The conclusions of
McCabe and those like him could only be defeated by the
incompatability of their analysis and the evidence of 'success' which
Latta and his followers might gather. Even these might be dismissed as
temporary relief, which they were in many instances, or as successes
due to other causes. Logical argument was not a process which could
decide the issue. In the end the doctor or scientist would have to transfer
belief from one system to another, helped by the *ad hominem* evidence
presented by people like Latta and Lewins.

Nor could the empirical evidence decide the issue. At Warrington 28
out of 30 patients recovered, at York only four out of 23.
Correspondents to the medical journals countered accounts of success
with accounts of failure. The failures tended to predominate. The
treatment was only carried out in hospital. Most patients only entered
hospital in the worst collapse stage of the disease and doctors only
used the new untried treatment in desperate cases. John Anderson,
surgeon, RN, on the convict ships at Rochester had a 'captive' group of
patients. He claimed that saline treatment started in the early stages of
the disease was almost certain of success.[21] At the end of May when
Christison and his fellows came to see the results of the treatment at the
Drummond Street hospital, the Professor was impressed by the fact that
25 out of 156 otherwise hopeless cases had been saved. The system was
worth a 'trial', but 'I am far from thinking that the results of this
remedy are fairly established.' He still wanted to restrict its use to the
worst cases because of the risk that air might enter the veins of the
patient or that the vein itself would be damaged. 'This is a material
difficulty which must be guarded against by careful attention on the
part of the operator.' Latta's treatment not only challenged scientific
tradition but made impossibly high demands on medical resources and
skilled manpower. Latta's description showed that he needed two
operators and an assistant to perform the operation safely and
successfully. Latta also demanded a perfect high quality syringe; Read's
patent one with a silver tube. He wanted the saline solution at a

controlled temperature, around 112°F.

Critics and supporters of the method could not have known that the preparation of the saline solution in non-sterile conditions and the frequent bacterial contamination consequent on this would have caused many cases of septicaemia. This probably accounts for the divergent experiences of success and failure with the treatment.[22] Most local boards of health found it difficult enough to supply a hospital, and pay the medical men to visit each case for a few minutes or so. Latta's treatment had to be ignored by most doctors and administrators because they had neither the time nor equipment to sustain the skilled attention to each patient which was demanded.

The saline treatment had to await considerable advances in medical technology, resources and understanding before it was adopted.

(iv) Etiology and Prevention

The advice which a doctor gave on the prevention of cholera depended on which theory he accepted on the spread of cholera. There were four different kinds of etiological theory. There was the religious explanation. Few men denied the Almighty some part in the epidemic, but most left a place for secondary causes.

Contagionist theory was the most widely accepted. It was the common-sense view. Cholera was communicated from person to person, from the sick to the healthy by direct personal contact. The *Lancet* gave a simple undramatic account,

> We can only suppose the existence of a poison which progresses independently of the wind, of the soil, of all conditions of the air and of the barrier of the sea; in short one that makes mankind the chief agent for its dissemination.

As one early Bengal report stated, it was 'a cause depending on communication with the diseased'.[23] Few discussed the nature of the poison, and only one man appeared to have attempted to link cholera with the 'animalacular' objects which some scientists had seen in their microscopes. Dr Adam Neale believed that disease was carried by clouds of minute insects too small for the eye to detect, helped along by favourable winds and an imbalance in terrestial electricity. Neale's insects had little in common with modern 'germs'; 'the minute insects commissioned by the DIVINE OMNIPOTENCE, to this end, are probably wafted in straight lines through the atmosphere'.[24] The failure of Neale and the orthodox contagionists to see that the 'poison' was a self-reproducing organism meant that their theory had only a superficial resemblance to modern germ theory.

The major rival to contagion theory attributed cholera to a non-contagious influence, frequently described as a vapour or miasma, which was spontaneously generated by a variety of localised causes. It 'springs from the bowels of the earth', said an Indian army surgeon, but the heaps of decaying vegetation and filth which accumulated in the streets of all cities from Calcutta to Sunderland attracted most attention. 'Morbific miasma', explained Whitelaw Ainslie, another Indian doctor, was 'bred and brewed, on the noisome face of a dark morass – within the confines and narrow lanes of a large, crowded, ill-ventilated city – on the ensanguined plain, amidst thousands of unburied dead. . .' Gaulter in Manchester realised that this 'unknown deleterious agent' acted on the alimentary canal. Henry Dodd, the local surgeon at Houghton-le-Spring, a growing mining township west of Sunderland, blamed the unseasonable weather and 'a column of pestilential matter arising in, or borne to certain districts, where it is attracted or detained by local causes hitherto unknown and undefined'.[25] Others blamed electric fluid, rising from the earth or from 'warm and damp (atmosphere). . .surcharged with electric fluid, it hence impairs the whole nervous system, but especially the ganglionic nerves'.[26]

Other theories, allied in some ways to the miasmatic, attributed cholera to some remote cause, often an extraordinary terrestial event. The *Lancet* rejects this as little better than the Highlander who blamed the fairies but gave a tolerant list.

> Baffled in these theories, the mind of man, ever prodigal in speculation, launched out new hypotheses in the utmost profusion. Mr. Orton spoke of negative, others of positive electricity. A third saw a comet in the east. A fourth marked the rise of a volcano. A fifth, Dr. Adam Neale, . . . heard a swarm of green flies in Astrakan and straight-way he jumped at his conclusion of the generation by animate contagion. A sixth attributed the malady to astronomical changes.[27]

Several doctors found the major theories inadequate and were fascinated by these strange notions. T. Forster of Boreham in Essex wrote of 'unusual and unwonted changes of heat and cold, of unwonted meteors, whirlwinds, waterspouts, fogs, etc. . .'. There was a new volcano reported off Sicily and a remarkable aurora borealis seen in the north of England.[28] Clanny spent his spare hours before the arrival of cholera

in Sunderland counting flashes of lightning, hoping to find a clue to
the causes of the disease. Adam Neale was even more apocalyptic. On
17 August a spectacular thunderstorm passed from Dover to Liverpool,

> a body of vapour of extraordinary magnitude, arising apparently out
> of the earth, accompanied by a very loud rumbling noise. It resembled
> the smoke of a conflagration and had a fiery appearance. It
> continued ascending for the space of about three minutes, all of the
> time accompanied by the noise above mentioned.[29]

Here, he thought, was the means by which Divine Providence had
disseminated those minute insects. The failure of the rational empirical
traditions of science allowed a more primitive thought pattern to
emerge. There was an archetypal fittingness in the correlation between
violent disruptions of nature, thunder, lightning and volcanoes, and the
violent disruption of the human body by cholera. It was a correspondence
of natural, social and personal events which would have satisfied the
readers of Aquinas and Shakespeare not just as analogy but as
explanation.

In 1832, the contagionist and non-contagionist systems of
explanations had the greatest social importance. Both theories were
present in the ancient world and medieval Europe. They were argued
over during the seventeenth-century London plagues, but by the
eighteenth century contagionist arguments had come to dominate
policy. Richard Mead based his quarantine policy on contagion in 1720.
As the major towns came to build general hospitals, they excluded
infectious disease like smallpox and syphilis from their wards. After
1800, contagionist explanations were being challenged with increasing
successes, especially by research designed to gain some relaxation of the
quarantine laws which hampered commerce.

The wide variety of preventative measures used were each derived
from one or both of these theories. Quarantine was clearly related to
contagion. 'A little commercial inconvenience is a small price to pay
for the chance of immunity,' said the *Edinburgh Medical and Surgical
Journal* at the start of the epidemic. But after the experience of the
autumn and winter of 1831, the *Journal* asked, 'Have they obtained any
object worth the immense expense and most serious interruption of
trade, commerce and general intercourse...what chance is there of such
a system being faithfully and effectually enforced in this land of
liberty'? The *Lancet* anticipated a 'civil contest' if attempts were made
to impose systematic internal quarantine.[30] Quarantine and contagion

were being discredited not on scientific grounds, but on social ones, by the inadequacy of administration and a value system which demanded freedom of movement. The other major implication of contagion was the isolation of the sick in cholera hospitals, which were built as much to stop the spread of the disease as to cure the sick. Here again, success was limited by the social response. The fear and resentment of the lower classes meant that entry to hospital had to be voluntary, thus limiting the effect of the policy.

Most local boards prepared for cholera with a programme of whitewashing and fumigation in the crowded and dirty parts of their area. Most official advice mentioned whitewash, hot lime wash or chloride of lime. Householders were advised to 'hot lime wash the walls of your house from cellar to garrett'. The Oxford Board made lime available to individuals so this could be done, and most boards poured large quantities into drains and sewers. The more systematic investigations of the twentieth century have shown that chloride of lime is a valuable disinfectant, especially when added to the water supply.[31] In 1832, large quantities of the right chemical were being used with an indiscriminate enthusiasm which must have left many channels of infection untouched.

In places as far apart as Exeter and Cromarty, fumigation was carried out in the most primitive manner by burning barrels of pitch and tar in the streets. In Oxford, the local board heard of the burning of tar barrels in the streets of Bristol, and resolved to order several to burn in Bull Street, then the centre of an explosive epidemic. Paisley had a fumigation in March. The bell-ringers gave the signal to begin. The doctors said it was no use, but as the Glasgow paper claimed 'it is better to do something...than to stand idly looking on while the enemy is thriving in our ranks.'[32] Fumigation with strong and foul-smelling agents was a traditional reaction to disease and plague. The Hindus burnt a resinous substance, and pitch and sulphur had appeared in Britain against the plague. The same basic principle of association operated between pitch, tar and cholera as between thunder, volcanoes and the disease. The violent assault upon life and health was countered by a substance which made a violent assault upon the senses. During the anxieties of the epidemic fumigation was direct evidence to everyone's sense of smell that something was being done. Noise also had a traditional part in warding off disease. Whilst the governors of Shiraz in Persia ordered salvoes of artillery from dawn to dusk and the people of India and China drove out cholera with drums and timbrels, the brass band at Partick paraded the streets each night, some said to cheer

people up, but others noted it had played the cholera out of town.[33]
The inhabitants of places filled with noise and smell must have felt that
this assault on their senses, reminiscent of tales of hell, was an effective
counter-terror to cholera. The small fishing village of Musselburgh took
measures as primitive as a rural Chinese village,

> The means by which the profession have employed here for preventing
> the infection spreading in the houses and apartments of those
> labouring under the disease, are, fumigation with the means already
> mentioned (he meant ventilation), with the addition of the fumes of
> nitric and muriatic acids, burning tar, turpentine, vinegar, fumes of
> tobacco, flashing gunpowder, throwing vinegar and spirits of camphor
> throughout the apartment.[34]

Fumigation like whitewash had its scientific as well as primitive side.
The Central Board of Health employed the leading chemist Faraday to
investigate the disinfecting qualities of chlorine gas, but he found little
evidence, which was inevitable, since he did not know what the chlorine
was supposed to be destroying.[35] Whitewash and fumigation were areas
of action where, in varying degrees, the promptings of tradition, of
contagion and miasmatic theories and the findings of modern science do
overlap in their recommendations.

Contagionists and non-contagionists were united by the concept of
predisposing causes in their support of many measures concerning
cleansing, diet and personal habits. All observers noted that exposure to
contagion or miasma did not automatically result in cholera, and a list
of predisposing causes was rapidly drawn up. The *Lancet* gave a fairly
full list,

> ...the history of these maladies furnishes abundant proof that a
> crowded population, poverty, filth, foul air, unwholesome food,
> especially bad water, depressing passions, habits of intemperance,
> defective clothing, and general bodily debility, powerfully predispose
> to the reception of these diseases, and increase their mortality when
> received...[36]

Henry Dodd's list concentrated more on personal qualities. Some
had a natural or inherited predisposition. Others acquired one by,

> grief, watching, fasting, want of cleanliness, innutricious and irregular
> diet, the depression which succeeds the excitement from drinking

ardent spirits, utero-gestation and parturition; in short, whatever produced diminished energy of the nervous system, and lessened vascular action to the surfaces.[37]

From India in 1819 to Wick in 1832 the list was very much the same, even in 1848-9 the Board of Health list was altered only by a change in emphasis from depressing passions to filth, poor drainage and other environmental conditions.[38]

It followed from this that prevention should include the removal of predisposing causes. Special attention was given to drink and diet. 'Repletion and indigestion should be guarded against; all raw vegetables, acescent, unwholesome food and drink avoided'. More homely advice came from the *Foreign Quarterly:* avoid 'exposure to cold, to chills, to the night dew, to wet and moisture; the use of cold fluids, and of cold, flatulent and unripe fruits...'[39] Others warned against cucumbers, fish and cabbages, and a number of food prejudices spread with the epidemic. The fall in the demand for salmon threatened to ruin the owners of several northern fisheries. Both medical and social experience provided good grounds for avoiding such foods. They were all associated with stomach upsets. This was especially important to those who believed that all stomach disorders had the same basic cause. Thus all ills of the stomach were regarded as potential cholera and best avoided. A good way to do this was to avoid fruit and vegetables. Modern interest in vitamins and nutrition means that vegetables and fresh fruit are regarded with great favour. In the nineteenth-century town they were looked on with great suspicion as unwashed, slightly rotten and potential carriers of disease, especially summer diarrhoea.

In many areas frantic campaigns were organised to remove filth from streets, drains and watercourses.

The Board of Health advised the burning of 'decayed rags, cordage, papers and old clothes' and 'the removal of all forms of filth'. As soon as the boards of health were formed in Exeter, in Leeds, in Edinburgh and Oxford, they organised various forms of inspection of their towns and began the removal of 'nuisances', the legal name for the heaps of rubbish and sewage. Leeds carted huge amounts of manure from the yards of Briggate. Exeter paid especial attention to the offal from slaughter-houses which was usually thrown on to the street. In Edinburgh, the Board of Health spent £280 on cleansing the narrow streets and closes of the old parts of the City. Thirty extra scavengers were employed and 3,000 extra cart-loads of rubbish carried away from houses and cellars as well as open spaces. After consulting the medical profession, the police and magistrates acted swiftly to eliminate the dwelling-house pigs which were chiefly kept by immigrant Irish who supplemented meagre wages by selling the flesh and dung.[40]

These efforts were too little and too late. No short-term programme could have been successful. Even the law was against the local boards. The task needed years of development, the organisation of scavengers and the building of systems of drainage and water supply. It was not the task of a few months.

(v) Contagion v. Miasma

Scientific standards gave the men of 1832 no clear guidance in choosing between the two major systems of explanation available. In many ways the structure of the debate fitted the Kuhnian model of the development of scientific thought.

There was no progressive and orderly accumulation of knowledge, but a heated debate between competing systems of explanation, which filled journals and pamphlets with claim and counter claim, often talking at cross purposes because they were observing different rules of scientific argument. The situation had many features of the pre-science phase of the Kuhnian model. Neither system gave a complete account of natural events. Neither gained complete acceptance from the scientific community – indeed, such a community hardly existed in the medical world of 1832. One reason for this was the lack of an authoritative paradigm to guide their thoughts and research. There was no agreement about the nature of the problem. There was no agreement about the terms and concepts in which the problem should be discussed – should it be miasmas or contagions or remote causes? There was no agreement about relevant evidence – should it be first contacts, or the correlation of dirt and disease on urban cholera maps? Characteristic of the pre-paradigm phase was the random collection of all kinds of evidence from Clanny watching the lightning over Sunderland to Robert Baker who recorded the swarm of black insects on a lady's washing in Leeds, and the men who studied humidity, the emergence of new volcanoes, and habits of diet and drink. The study of any one class of natural events only enters a purposeful scientific phase when a paradigm has been developed and accepted. The paradigm is a fundamental scientific achievement, often embodied in one of the great standard works of a subject, like Newton's *Principia*, Lyell's *Geology* or Franklin's *Electricity*. These works embodied theory and some practical demonstration of that theory, but were more than this. It gained unequivocal and binding authority over the minds of the scientific community which formed around it and excluded all other sorts of explanation from their minds. The paradigm told the scientist about relationships between natural events. It also told him what sort of things to talk about, what experimental methods, what concepts and observations were relevant in the discussion of similar problems. There then followed a period of normal science, of problem-solving, as when the methods of Pasteur and Koch were systematically applied to other diseases at the end of the nineteenth century. The authority of a paradigm was only broken when it became impossible to fit a number of important anomalies into the evidence. There then followed a scientific revolution in which the paradigm was adapted or replaced. This period bore some resemblance to the pre-scientific phase.

The cholera debate of 1832 had many characteristics of this revolutionary situation. The long-established, fairly widely accepted contagionist paradigm was being overthrown by miasmatic thinking in the light of anomalies revealed by diseases like cholera. The mixture of revolutionary and pre-paradigm features in one situation derived from the special nature of medical research as a science which answers immediate social needs. The answers to the day-to-day problems facing the doctor in his rounds must derive from a body of organised knowledge which has many of the features of the paradigm. It must be all-embracing, exclude all other systems and have the authority of acceptance from a significant section of the profession. The medical man was unable to ask his patient to wait awhile until science had developed a suitable paradigm. Authoritative advice was needed at once. Hence the attractions of the eighteenth-century systems, which gave an immediate and approved answer to all medical problems. Hence the bitterness and cross purposes with which the contagion/non-contagion debate was argued in the first half of the nineteenth century. Each doctor needed final and exclusive authority for his answers, for they concerned the life, death and fees of his patients. The contagion/non-contagion debate was less a debate between schools of thought than between competing paradigms, because of the claims to scientific authority made by supporters of both theories.[41] Contagion and miasma were more than just explanations. The use of either concept implied a whole system of thought and investigation which showed the researcher what to look for as well as what was significant. In this way the systems tended to be self-supporting, for they naturally drew attention to the sorts of evidence and interpretation of that evidence which confirmed the ability of the central concepts to explain events.

The task of a scientific community was and is to extend the range of natural events which can be explained by universally recognised knowledge. These explanations must be empirically confirmed and logically consistent. Scientific findings are communal property, to be published and not kept secret like a commercial patent. The doctors of 1832 did seek wider recognition by publishing their findings and exposing them to the critical appraisal of their fellows. Ideally, if scientific knowledge claims to be universal, these findings ought to be accepted or rejected without regard to the status of the researcher whether this be in terms of birth, income, seniority or prestige. Nor should research be guided by any other interest except the standards of scientific debate. In practice, these two standards are hard to achieve. In 1832, they were nearly impossible. The government sought the advice of the Royal College of Physicians because of their prestige. London discoveries and claims tended to gain more attention in the journals than provincial ones. Many of Latta's problems derived from his social position, not the scientific problems raised by his method. Many doctors found miasmatic theory compatible with their place in a commercial community.

The men who wrote the cholera literature of 1832 did not talk in terms of a scientific community, indeed they preferred the more gentlemanly term natural philosopher to that of scientist. Concern for the values of such a community was expressed in the continual references back to the basic principles of cause and effect which appear as part of otherwise very specific writing about cholera. This looking back to first principles is always a feature of scientific debate which lacks an authoritative paradigm. In the medical world of 1832, especially in Scotland, discussing the first principles of human knowledge and of cause and effect meant going back to David Hume. The *Glasgow Medical Journal* quoted directly, 'We can never be allowed to ascribe to the cause any qualities, but what are exactly sufficient to produce the effect.'

In the early days the *Lancet* found that 'multiplied coincidences are tantamount to actual demonstration', and decided for contagion, but David Craigie criticised such methodology. 'Coincidence in time and place', he wrote, 'it cannot be too frequently repeated, do not positively indicate the relation of cause and effect.' Gaulter made the same point as he prepared to demolish the contagionist position.[42]

In the face of such arguments and without the authority and guidance of a paradigm none of the evidence produced could have led to any conclusion. A full account of the evidence was given in all the medical periodicals. The contagionists could show that cholera followed lines of human communication across Europe; trade routes, armies in Poland and Russia, pilgrims in Bombay and Mecca. It had come with the frigate *Topaz* to Mauritius and been brought by a Russian brig to Baku. When cholera reached Britain the first cases in each town and village were scrutinised with especial care to discover contact with infected places. The visit of the rag dealer Denis M'Guire made North Shields a good case for the contagionists, as were the German broomsellers in Dudley, but Haddington was victory for the anti-contagionists for the three shoemakers seemed to have arrived from Newcastle the day after cholera. The anti-contagionists pointed out that cholera did not spread in an even and continuous manner. It paused in winter. It missed out whole areas, and might jump without contact, as it had moved across the North Sea to Sunderland, and across Scotland to Kirkintilloch and Glasgow. In neither place could contact with infection be traced. The research continued with attempts to trace contacts within towns. The first 50 cases in Sunderland, and the first 200 in Manchester were closely followed. Some writers noted how often cholera spread in families; others noted how often it did not.[43] Quarantine itself was a practical test of both theories. The Cadet School at Cronstadt, the French Consul at Aleppo, the barracks at Sunderland all showed the validity of contagionist thinking, but the epidemic in the Town's Hospital at Glasgow attributed to the spontaneous generation of cholera in a nearby dunghill and the general failure of European quarantine showed that contact was not necessary.[44] Many doctors who started the epidemic as contagionists were convinced that they were wrong because they believed that doctors and nurses working with cholera patients did not catch the disease in the way they tended to do in epidemics like typhus. The doctors may have felt they escaped but they were selecting evidence and ignored a long list of dead among nurses and medical men. Four nurses died in Glasgow; eight in the Swan Street Hospital in Manchester. This could be attributed to the drunken and dissolute habits of many nurses at that time, but Mr Caird, surgeon in Musselburgh, died, as did four in Dumfries and thirteen in Sligo.[45] Although the medical profession suffered a greater cholera death rate than any other middle-class occupation, they were probably safer from this water-borne infection than from droplet infections.

During the epidemic, many doctors had been contagionist whilst looking at the map of Europe. Men like Harry Leake Gibbs, first surgeon at the naval hospital in St Petersburg, David Craigie visiting Newburn from Edinburgh, Lawrie and Molinson in north-east England, became anti-contagionist when they became deeply involved in the study and treatment of cholera in one location. Close attention to detail produced an unacceptable number of anomalies for contagionist analysis and they turned to other aspects of the evidence. After his visit to Newcastle Lawrie wrote that cholera preferred low-lying, densely populated, filthy areas. Gaulter came to the same conclusion in Manchester. The cause was miasma spontaneously generated in such areas. Baker mapped the cases in Leeds and showed the same 'cholera geography'. The contagionist accounted for this by suggesting that as the rate of human contact was greater in areas of dense population so the rate of infection was greater. He also warned that the inability to trace contacts did not mean that the contact did not exist. Filth and crowding were 'predisposing' causes when infection came, and not an effective cause on its own, besides the filth had been there long before the cholera. This sent the miasmatic men searching for predisposing causes of their own, in individual behaviour and in the humidity and electricity in the atmosphere. Most of the evidence could be accounted for in terms of either paradigm and hence scientific rules, careful empirical observation, rigorous consistency of reasoning, and the powerful principles of induction and association were unable to resolve the debate. Perhaps in the scientific conditions of 1832, the Westminster Medical Society were right when they decided the matter by open vote.[46]

Because the choice between the two paradigms could not be made by scientific rules, the choice was directed by social pressures from outside the medical community. This was possible because of the lack of assurance, and the lack of a sophisticated, authoritative logical structure on the part of medical science. It did not have its own concepts, procedures and forms of debate, features which enable so many scientific discussions to be conducted in the public domain of articles, lectures and reports and yet retain an exclusiveness and privacy which derives from the inaccessibility of language, concepts and traditions to all but the specially trained and initiated. Medical discussions in 1832 continually had to return to the basic tasks of description and elementary reasoning. The refuge of the Latinate terms of *materia medica* gave the doctor very little cover from social pressures. By its very nature medical science provided most groups in society with some motive for paying attention to its activities. Everyone is and was a potential patient, a potential subject for medical research. Most are liable to public health regulations.

Although British social action and opinion was dominated by

contagionist thinking in 1831, anti-contagionist views gained increasing favour as the epidemic spread. John Lizars welcomed the conversion of many medical men who worked in or visited north-east England in November 1831. The trend of opinion was the same in London in March 1832. The Westminster Medical Society had three anti-contagionists in November 1831. When they took their vote, the majority was against contagion. British medical thought had begun to doubt the contagious nature of many diseases. The intensity of discussion on cholera in 1832 highlighted the identity of the social groups which supported each side of the debate. The swing of opinion was not only part of a scientific debate, but also a result of key social groups asserting their influence on British opinion and policy.

In the early wave of books and pamphlets written about the approaching cholera, those who visited Russia or read the reports from there tended to be contagionist, whilst the medical men with Indian experience tended to be against contagion. J.H. Kennedy, one of the few contagionists to come from India had, according to James Johnson, only 37 other medical men who supported him in the rest of India.[47] Of the three Presidency reports prepared after the 1818 epidemic, two were contagionist and only Calcutta reported for miasma, but over the following decade the books and articles from India almost all denied contagion. When the Central Board of Health interviewed six Indian medical men in the summer of 1831, four of them claimed cholera was not contagious and two said the evidence was conflicting. The only contagionist witness was Count Michael Waronzow, Governor of Odessa during the cholera epidemic in that province. The bulk of writing by men with Indian experience, which was reviewed in 1831-2, was anti-contagion; George Hamilton Bell, *Treatis on Cholera Asphyxia;* J.A. Lawrie, *Essays on cholera. . .in Sunderland. . .;* Reginald Orton, *Essay on the Epidemic Cholera of India,* London, 1830; T. Mollison, *Remarks on the Cholera as it occurred in Newcastle,* were all in this group. James Annesley was something of an exception. Indian experience made him an anti-contagion man but a study of European evidence converted him against the tide of opinion to the more traditional view. Now most of the men named were also surgeons, who were of lower social status than the physicians, and most were or had been army surgeons who were of lower social status than those with general or hospital practice. Of those surgeons from the English towns who went into print after and during 1831-2, most were also anti-contagionist, T.W. Greenhow from North Shields, White from Gateshead, Dodd from Houghton-le-Spring, Gaulter in Manchester and Baker in

Leeds, although some like Ogier Ward in Wolverhampton were as firmly contagionist. The authorities in the Scottish universities also tended to be anti-contagion, in Glasgow more so than Edinburgh – the *Edinburgh Medical and Surgical Journal* never completely rejected the doctrine which many of its contributors attacked and which the *Glasgow Medical Journal* rejected from the start. The authorities of London, from the Royal College of Physicians to the *Lancet,* all began, and some finished, as contagionists. Thus the lower-status groups in the medical profession, men from the middle classes but who shared little of the authority of government, the India men, the surgeons, and the Scots all tended to go into print as anti-contagionists.

The commercial elements of the middle class gave a natural welcome to the anti-contagion trend and their part in the political opposition to and defeat of contagion has already been discussed.

In other men, medical and scientific judgement was influenced by moral considerations. John Goss left a suspicion in his writing that he rejected contagion, not only on scientific grounds, doctors and people on high ground escaped, contacts could not be traced, but also because the fears contagion produced prevented people doing their 'moral duty' to the sick. James Johnson was another who warmly advocated miasma on social grounds. Without contagion there would be no disruption of trade, with lost jobs and profits, no fear of the sick, and no excuse for dragging working-class patients off to hospital with all the attendant discontent. John Lizars suggested that, in addition, contagionist doctrine reduced the moral effects which cholera was intended to have. Many predisposing causes emphasised moral behaviour but if contagion was accepted,

> The minds of the vicious are lulled into fatal security; so long as the drunkard avoids the infected district, he considers himself beyond its influence; and in desperation, consoles himself in the certainty of his escape, and halts not in his reckless revelries.

The manner in which Lizars elaborates his position suggests that there was a particular compatibility between evangelical and miasmatic thinking.

> Had the public therefore in place of being terrified by the bugbear of contagion, been warned by the same authorities, of this undisputed fact, that cholera is epidemic – that it had been cast upon us by the inscrutable workings of Divine Providence, which no human power

can avert; and that no man could tell who would be affected and
who would escape, the same precautions as to health, temperance,
cleanliness and attention to the wants of the poor, would have been
observed.[48]

Miasmatic doctrines enabled the evangelical to regard cholera more
fatalistically – not the fatalism of inaction, but the fatalism of trust in
God whilst leading a Christian life. Under a non-contagionist system the
incidence of cholera was far more unpredictable than under contagion,
hence more room was left for Divine intervention.

The social groups which identified with contagionist views can be
more readily identified with social classes. Contagion was a ruling-class
doctrine. It was part of the administrative memory of the plague and
the advice of Richard Mead, confirmed by Select Committee of
Parliament, upheld by Russell and Barry, given further authority by the
Royal College of Physicians and defended in pamphlet form by the
Board of Health and by Sir Henry Halford. Contagion was the doctrine
of strong government. The rules and regulations which derived from the
doctrine enabled government to seize more authority than they could
have done under miasmatic theory. Government could disrupt trade,
confine people to hospital, create panic which might divert attention
from reform. Contagion brought specific executive action whilst miasma
implied few short-term measures, although the middle classes were to
find that the government claimed considerable power of property when
the longer-term implications of miasma became clear.

There was no highly developed working-class view on etiology. Some,
like *Carpenter's,* suspected contagion because of its links with ruling-class
action. Others like the *Poor Man's Guardian* and *Cobbett's Journal*
followed the contagionist line on common-sense grounds, suspecting in
their turn the motives of the commercial lobby. There were some
elements of the aristocratic-working-class alliance which included a
sharing of views on sport and drinking habits, and which was to appear
in the political alliance which helped the Factory Acts on to the statute
book. It was natural that the working class, with few facilities and little
organisation for developing their own views on cholera, should accept
fairly readily the dominant opinion and favour contagion.

The miasmatic view did not identify readily with a middle class of
any sort. Most middle-class people accepted the dominant view as
readily as the rest of the country, but surgeons, army and India men,
and Scots doctors, elements of the middle class, did tend to miasma. By
1848-9, miasma had come to dominate government thinking. It did so

as middle-class influence began to take a greater part in government through the new urban franchise of 1832. Its main propagandist was Edwin Chadwick, riding on the back of the bourgeois empirical tradition of Benthamite Utilitarianism. Chadwick himself was to fail because he ignored and treated with contempt the power base of the middle class whose ideas he represented, the local authorities and communities who would have to pay the rates for public health measures.

The identity of contagionist and miasmatic views with particular social groups and classes was not a deterministic one. There were Indian medical men who accepted contagion. There were commercial men who did likewise. Even in autocratic Russia, firmly identified with contagion and strong government, the authorities followed European opinion in the next epidemic and accepted miasmatic views. Social and moral views were important in forming opinions on scientific matters in 1832, but the logic of scientific argument and tradition still had a major part to play. To borrow the language of the cholera debate itself, social and moral pressures did not determine views on cholera but they were important predisposing conditions.

(vi) Limitations and Methods of Medical Research

The debate was confused and open to social and moral pressure because it took place without any acknowledgement of its central character, the *cholera vibrio,* or even a partial knowledge of the manner in which it spread. Social and moral pressure, and the inadequacies of scientific tradition could not, on their own, be responsible for this failure. The disregard and poor development of statistics and the limitations of the microscope set formidable technical barriers to research.

The microscope for scientific research had been developed in the late sixteenth and seventeenth centuries. One of its most skilled users, the Dutchman Leeuwenhook, was the first man to see and record bacteria – 'wee animals' – on the human tooth. An eighteenth-century knowledge of 'wonderfully minute living creatures' seen through the microscope kept alive a theory of *contagium animatum.* But the microscopes available up to 1832 had two major defects, chromatic and spherical aberration. Before the work of J.J. Lister in London and the Chevaliers in Paris between 1824 and 1830, any image at high magnification was seen in a halo of coloured light which blurred the edges of small objects. Coupled with the effects of spherical aberration, this meant that small objects appeared to be globular or fibrillar. During the eighteenth century whole systems of natural philosophy were based upon these distorted observations, thus adding to the general distrust which men like Linnaeus had for the instrument. Lister's work produced clearer images but the microscope did not become a regular part of medical research and education until Quekett introduced it to London in the 1840s. Until that date medical research had made no consistent use of the microscope because adequate instruments were not available. The only mention of the microscope in the 1832 cholera literature comes in the *Lancet* survey which makes it clear that some of the Broussian school, the ideologists, used a microscope in their autopsies to study the damage done to the organs and tissues, not to look for minute living organisms. Neale, the leading pamphleteer of the animalcular wing of the contagionist school, realised that the microscope might help his case, made a reference to Leeuwenhook, but gives no indication that he ever used one himself. Cholera came a generation too soon for the *vibrio* to be identified and studied.[49]

The greatest volume of cholera literature was an endless stream of case histories contained in dozens of pamphlets and hundreds of letters, notes and articles in the medical Press. All followed the same pattern, details of symptoms and the results of varied forms of treatment. A few of these histories finished with details of post-mortems, despite the denials which were issued to crowds which threatened riot and destruction. In the winter of 1831, Professor Delpech visited lowland Scotland and on his visit to Musselburgh took advantage 'of the permission we had received of inspecting the bodies of such as should fall victims to the disease'. He did this with such thoroughness in Glasgow and along the Forth that he was able to give detailed descriptions of the internal damage done by cholera. Lizars, who published this work, was able to base his own writing on twenty dissections which he had carried out in the centre of the area troubled by riots over just this issue. From the evidence he gathered he concluded that cholera resulted in wholesale failure of the nervous system. Down in Leith, Latta also resorted to post-mortem investigation to find why cases treated by the saline method did on occasion die.[50]

The readers of these case histories could have learnt little except perhaps that their own failure was reflected in the work of others, or that a new technique had brief success and might replace their own. Systematic analysis of these reports was impossible because no one attempted a comparative analysis of the success of the different methods. Statistical tables were few. Most concerned death case ratios or the ages of those who died; only a few, like the letter to the *London Medical Gazette* from Warrington, gave percentage recoveries for different methods of treatment, and these got little recognition from other writers. Statistics was not an accepted technique for validating the findings of medical science. Like the microscope, the statistical movement was to develop a decade too late to help the analysis of information collected in 1832.

What did develop in 1832 was the medical community study. This grew from the medical topography of the eighteenth century which was 'that science which teaches the effects of climate, locality, and other external circumstances upon health'. Sydenham had a general interest in the relationship between disease and locality but this had become more systematic under two influences, the general topographies inspired by Camden and Stukeley and then the interest in the classification and distribution of plants which the medical profession gained from Linnaeus. They were closely linked to botany through the herbalists.[51]

After 1832, there were a small number of detailed studies which related the distribution of cholera to the environment and social relationships of the victims and their community. These studies included Baker on Leeds, Gaulter on Manchester, Haslewood and Mordey in Sunderland, and in a more limited way the writing of Vaughan-Thomas in Oxford and Girdlestone and Leigh in the Black Country. It was a form of parasociology which gave rise to the statistical movement, and to the subsequent studies of poverty, crime and education which led to the work of Mayhew, Booth and the parliamentary commissions later in the century and laid the groundwork for the empirical community-based studies which form a major part of British sociology today.

These local studies were made by members of the two professions which provided a link between the working classes and the classes above them, namely the ministers of religion and the medical profession. The two Black Country parsons, Leigh and Girdlestone, related the cholera with moral and social behaviour. They were remarkable for seeing moral faults and cholera — both of which were condemned, against the background of social and economic conditions. Moral failings like drunkenness were presented as part of local work and recreational patterns, and not subjected to the disembodied case by case censure of the Methodist, or to the abstract criticism of the fast day sermon. James Kay's report on Manchester had the same concern plus the backing of medical experience. He related drinking habits to the harshness and tedium of workplace and living conditions, and in turn related disease and poverty to drinking habits. Vaughan-Thomas, vicar of Yarnton and chairman of the Oxford Board of Health, a more traditionalist churchman than those mentioned above, widened his analysis and related the disease to bad drainage, crowded housing, lack of ventilation, dirty streets and the 'destitute state of the poor', in a manner that would have done credit to any of the miasmatist doctors.

The cholera experience tempted many obscure medical men into print with detailed accounts of their locality. Thomas Proudfoot had already produced a medical topography of Kendal and in 1832 used the same methods to study cholera. He believed that the 'united efforts of many observers' were needed to solve the problem of how cholera spread and evidently felt he was contributing a small piece to a much greater enterprise. Much of his account was an ordinary medical report of case histories and treatment. Indeed, several of the local reports, like James Alderson in Hull and Ogier Ward at Wolverhampton, are little more than this and never developed into a true community study. Proudfoot began to relate the disease to local conditions when he became interested in the housing conditions of his patients. In his investigations of Robinson's Close he came very near the truth. Six of the 96 inhabitants of the Yard died. Water supply came from a pump well half way up the yard. At the top of the yard the houses were joined by privies with a 'dunghill of the most revolting description' in the ground floor of a nearby house – in which lived one of the cholera families, 'From the dunghill and the privies there is every reason to believe that moisture percolated the earth, and vitiated the water in the well. . .'. He was then diverted by the observation that cholera rarely appeared twice in the same family and hence after a case-by-case enquiry which discovered no contact between the cases, he concluded that the disease was not infectious.

The best of the community studies came from the medical profession, for they were designed to answer the question, was cholera spread by contact between people, or was it not? Haslewood and Mordey began their survey of the epidemic in Sunderland with a description of local topography and occupations, pointing out the effect of delays in the arrival of shipping which brought the sailors, porters and others linked with the port to poverty and the pawnshop. Their main interest was tracing contacts, so they constructed a table, case by case, showing name, residence and trade, sex, whether died or lived and other 'remarks' which included drinking habits and contact with other cases. As a result of this they concluded against the tide of opinion that the disease was most likely contagious, but agreed that it could be spread by other means, and had most likely arrived in Sunderland as a miasma.

Table 12: *Tabular view*, showing Connection between the Subjects of Attacks of Cholera, which came under the Notice of the Authors

Date of Attack	No.	Name	Residence and Trade	Sex	Event	Remarks
Oct. 23	1	Sproat, Senior	On the Quay, Labourer	M	Died	No contagion has been traced: he laboured under diarrhoea and other disorders for some days previous to the attack. Attended by Mr. Holmes, Surgeon
27	2	Sproat, Junior	Ballast Keelman	M	Died	Communicated with No. 1, his father; died in the Infirmary
—	3	Sproat	—	F	Recovered	Daughter of No. 2 Infirmary
31	4	Rodenby	Quay, Monk Wearmouth, Shoemaker	M	Died	No connection traced
—	5	Thomas Wilson	High Street, Keelman	M	Died	No connection traced
Nov. 1	6	Nurse	Infirmary	F	Died	Assisted in removing the body of No. 2, but did not see him during life: she was under great alarm, and was attacked some hours afterwards.
6	7	Etherington	Burleigh Street, Sailor	M	Died	Had been in a weak state for some time previous; died the same day
—	8	Ellimore	Hatcase, Pilot	M	Died	Was an habitual drunkard; was very drunk the day previous

Source: W. Haslewood and W. Mordey, *The History and Medical Treatment of Cholera as it appeared in Sunderland in 1831*, London, 1832, pp. 124-5.

David Craigie presented his information from Newburn in a similar manner but he concentrated more on place and type of residence and less on occupation and contacts. His results were more firmly in favour of miasmatic or spontaneous generation of cholera. In Leeds, Robert Baker gathered and presented his information in a street by street survey. This method inevitably pointed to a relationship betweel local conditions and cholera, and could only have been chosen by an investigator who already favoured such a link. Medical topography as a *genre* was increasingly developed in a manner which favoured non-contagionist arguments.

Despite the careful presentation of evidence none of the tables attempted an analysis more sophisticated than correlation by inspection. Not even a frequency distribution was prepared for any of the variables included in the table. The factor which prevented a fair evaluation of Latta's saline method of treatment operated to limit the effectiveness of the community studies; the medical profession did not use or have available the descriptive statistical techniques which were to be developed and accepted over the following decade.

Henry Gaulter was a firm supporter of the miasmatic paradigm. His study of Manchester was one of the most thorough and closely argued of the community studies. He surveyed local conditions and topography and gave a case-by-case presentation of his enquiry in the familiar tables. Gaulter was also the most explicit about the problems of collecting the information he wanted. His introduction was an impromptu manual on questionnaire technique in the conditions of 1832.

> The investigation of these causes (those by which the disease spread) cannot be successfully conducted without both trouble and address. Little information can be obtained from the patient himself, if he be not seen early, or after recovery; nor is it amidst the anxieties and painful excitement of a Cholera hospital, where the first and only consideration is, what can be done for the sufferer, that the facts which bear upon the history of the disease can be ascertained. The poor, too, are habitually inexact: they omit, from stupidity, the most essential point of an inquiry, unless led to it by a direct question; or they answer as they suppose you wish them to answer; or else they wilfully deceive; nor is it difficult to imagine many powerful motives for concealment or falsehood in such an investigation. It is often, in short, only by a separate examination and cross-examination of the patient, relations, and neighbours, managed with all the astuteness of a lawyer, and that too, after the

first alarm has passed away and the tranquillity of the house or
neighbourhood has been restored, that the true particulars of the
origin of any individual case can be correctly learned. Nor are the
poor the only deceivers. The inquirer is himself, from an unconscious
bias, not seldom in pursuit less of the truth whatever it may be and
wherever it may lead, than of some preconceived opinion or exclusive
system. He is a contagionist, and puts but one kind of question, or
hears but one class of answers: he is an adversary to contagion, and
interrogates only on localities and miasma.

The enquirer was hampered by suspicion between the authorities and
the poor, between the medical profession and the lower classes. He was
divided from his sources of information by cultural barriers which were
impossible to cross in the haste and tension of the epidemic. An honest
and reflective man like Gaulter knew that the paradigm which guided
his researches framed his questions in a way which sought the answers
that supported the paradigm he initially believed in, so that despite his
hours of hard work the results of the enquiry were neither impartial nor
objective.[52]

As the traditional methods of medical enquiry failed, the doctors
introduced the concepts and methods of chemical and electrical studies
in an attempt to break the deadlock. Both these areas of science had
developed rapidly in the sixty or seventy years before 1832. The
techniques of exact analysis used by the chemists showed their value in
the work of O'Shaughnessy which, by its exact account of the various
materials in the blood, led Latta to his saline treatment. Others used the
chemical analysis less productively to search for miasma and contagious
poison in the atmosphere. The mysteries of electricity, which was
occasionally used in galvanic treatment, held an even greater fascination
for the medical men. In Edinburgh, Whitelaw Ainslie read with care
Charles Wilkinson's *Elements of Galvanism* to find explanations for
what he knew of the clinical history of cholera. He believed that the
action of cholera produced acrimonious acid in the bowels, and that in
certain circumstances electricity could do the same. He knew from the
work of Priestley that lightning and electricity were the same, and so
concluded that the cholera was caused by an irregular or perverted flow
of electric fluid, perhaps associated with the flashes of lightning often
witnessed before an epidemic.[53] Many medical writers identified the
active principle of the nervous system with electricity. It was thus
natural to associate cholera with electricity as the disease produced
muscular spasms and was associated with a failure of the nervous

system.[54] Adam Neale watched his electroscope carefully and claimed that an abnormal negative charge in the atmosphere not only deprived the body of nervous and muscular power but encouraged the abundance of insect life.[55] Whitelaw Ainslie associated cholera and electricity together because both were unpredictable. He felt that the electricity of the lightning flash was the special means by which the Creator controlled what was going on in the atmosphere.

Scientific developments which were in the mainstream of physics diverted research into a byway of medical science where the anger of God still rode on the thundercloud. The *Monthly Reivew*, casting a layman's eye over the literature, summed this meeting of ancient and modern perceptions in a phrase which united medieval imagery with the cool reasoning of Faraday's workbench, '. . .it must appear as if we were all but so many links of an electric chain descending from Heaven to the remotest material objects of the whole creation'.[56]

So, in 1832, the medical and scientific community failed to produce an adequate account of cholera, and failed to reach an understanding complete enough to produce effective preventative measures and cures. They failed despite the devotion of many hours of their time and inches of print to fact-gathering, exposition and argument. Two main types of enquiry were conducted. There was the study of etiology by the miasmatic and contagionist schools with occasional incursion of lesser themes. The bulk of substantive research into this question was done by provincial general practitioners. The best of them, like Gaulter and Baker, followed the model set by the medical topographers, and developed this towards the statistical presentation of social and medical information that was to continue in the 1830s. The results of their work circulated through local networks. Baker's was summarised in local papers and considered by the town council. Some of it was published in the provincial medical journals. These pamphlets got little notice in the London and Edinburgh medical journals. The other major type of enquiry concerned the pathology and clinical history of the disease. This was studied through countless case histories and autopsies. The pages of the medical journals and pamphlets were filled with symptoms, treatments, reactions, with meticulous detail on the state of each organ after death. This activity was led and largely carried out by the leading surgeons and physicians of the London and provincial hospitals. It was widely reported and discussed in all the leading medical journals. It led nowhere except to more confusion. Yet dissecting and prescribing were the most prestigious types of medical activity in 1832. The main base for medical research was in the hospitals of London and Edinburgh.

Here the anatomy theatre was the centre of teaching and the surgeon the hero of the organisation. In both centres the physician was the aristocrat of the profession, collecting large fees from giving advice to government, and orders to the rest of his calling. It was natural that most practitioners in the provinces should follow the models of enquiry set out and admired and rewarded above all others in medicine. Prestige, or the honour and reward granted to one type of activity or position over others, was a guiding factor in the choice of research model and interest, just as it is with many other social choices. The situation in 1832 was that the most prestigious means of enquiry were blocked by technical means. Microscopes were inadequate and statistical presentation little developed and less accepted. And the most effective form of enquiry in existing technical conditions, into etiology, was blocked by its lack of prestige. It was blocked by the most effective sanction the leaders and the media of any scientific community, or any other social group, can impose upon low-status minority groups in their ranks. Etiology was largely ignored and was given no help in terms of research facilities or resources.

From the lightning over Sunderland to the grim record of the dead-house in Glasgow, through the glimmer of truth in the ignored writing of Latta and Proudfoot; to the inadequacies of microscopes and statistics, and the tangled web of status and ambition which was the medical profession, the *cholera vibrio* escaped, undetected.

Notes

1. B. Hamilton, 'The Medical Profession in the 18th century', *Economic History Review*, 2nd series, vol.4, 1951. pp.141-69; S.W.F. Holloway, 'Medical Education in England, 1830-1858', *History*, vol.49, 1964, pp.299-324, and 'The Apothecaries Act, 1815', *Medical History*, vol.10, 1966, pp.221-30; William H. McMenemey, *The Life and Times of Sir Charles Hastings*, Edinburgh, 1959; 'Medical Reform'. *The Quarterly Review*, vol.67, 1841, pp.53-65.
2. *Poor Man's Guardian*, 30 March 1832.
3. Kenny Meadows, *Heads of the People*, London, c.1840, pp.57-64.
4. *New Monthly Magazine*, vol.34, 1832, p.296; *Poor Man's Advocate*, 25 February 1832.
5. *The Loyal Reformer's Gazette*, 25 February 1832.
6. *The British Critic*, vol.11, 1832, p.375; *The Wesleyan Methodist Magazine*, 1832, p.274.
7. *Edinburgh Evening Courant*, 17 March 1832.
8. Note dated December 1831 in P.C.1/103; Alison, Edinburgh, 21 November 1832 to MacLean, P.C.1/103; Arthur to MacLean, 3 May 1832, P.C.1/107; J. Barles, Airdrie, 5 April 1832, P.C.1/107, all in P.R.O.
9. R.H. Shryock, 'Nineteenth Century Medicine: scientific aspects', *Cahier*

Medicine and Science 193

d'histoire Mondiale, vol.3, 1957, pp.881-907.
10. George Hamilton Bell, *Treatis on the Cholera Asphyxia...*, Edinburgh, 1831; *Lancet*, 25 December 1830.
11. Whitelaw Ainslie, *Letters on Cholera*, London, 1832.
12. *Lancet*, vol.II, 1832, p.50.
13. *Lancet*, vol.II, 1832, p.797.
14. *E.M.S.J.*, vol.15, 1819, p.361; W. Ainslie, *Letters on Cholera*.
15. R.H. Shryock, *Cahier d'histoire Mondiale*, vol.3, 1957; George Rosen, 'The philosophy of Ideology and the emergence of modern medicine in France', *Bulletin of the History of Medicine*, vol.20, 1946, pp.329 ff.
16. *E.M.S.J.*, vol.37, 1832, p.207; *Lancet*, 19 November 1831, p.279; *Tait's Edinburgh Magazine*, vol.1, 1832.
17. *Lancet*, 1831-2, vol.I, p.490; Rough Minutes of the Central Board of Health, December 1831, P.R.O., P.C.1/105; Letter Book of the Central Board of Health, 31 May 1832, P.R.O., P.C.1/95; *Medical Gazette*, vol.10, p.20.
18. E.D.W. Grieg, 'The treatment of cholera by intra-venous saline injections, with particular reference to the contribution of Dr. Thomas Latta of Leith (1832)', *Edinburgh Medical Journal*, vol.53, 1946, pp.256-63; *Lancet*, vol.I, 1832, pp.173-6, 188 and 208; *Medical Gazette*, vol.10, p.257; Alastair H.B. Masson, 'Dr. Thomas Latta', *The Book of the Old Edinburgh Club*, vol.33, 1972, pp.143-9.
19. Robert Lewins to Dr MacLean, private letter explaining the circumstances of Dr Latta's work, written sometime in April or early May 1832, P.R.O., P.C.1/103.
20. Manuscript from James McCabe of Cheltenham, P.R.O., P.C.1/103.
21. *Lancet*, 1832, vol.II, p.78; James Alderson, *A brief outline of the history and progress of the cholera at Hull...*, London, 1832, pp.36-7; Note from John Anderson, M.C., surgeon RN to the Central Board of Health, P.R.O., P.C.1/103.
22. Robert Lewins to Dr MacLean, 29 May 1832 and Dr Christison to MacLean, 9 June 1832, P.R.O., P.C.1/103; Dr Christison, 'On the new treatment of cholera', *Medical Gazette*, vol.10, 1832, pp.451-2; 'Letter from Dr. Latta...', *Lancet*, vol.II, 1831-2, p.274; N. Howard-Jones, 'Cholera Therapy in the 19th century', *Journal of History of Medicine*, vol.27, 1972, pp.373-95.
23. Edward Alison, Edinburgh, 21 November 1831, to Mr MacLean, Central Board of Health, P.R.O. P.C.1/103; *Lancet*, 19 November 1832, p.261; *E.M.S.J.*, vol.16, 1820, p.460.
24. Adam Neale, *Researches to establish the truth of the Linnaean Doctrine of Animate Contagions...*, London, 1832, pp.5-7 and 232.
25. *Lancet*, 1832, vol.II, p.796.
26. John Lizars, *Substance of Investigations regarding Cholera Asphyxia in 1832...to which are added observations of the disease in Edinburgh*, Edinburgh, no date, pp.50-60.
27. *Lancet*, 19 November 1831.
28. *Lancet*, 22 October 1831.
29. Adam Neale, *Linnaean Doctrine of Animate Contagions*, p.237.
30. *E.M.S.J.*, vol.36, 1831, pp.139 and 404; *Lancet*, 19 November 1831, p.281.
31. Pollitzer, *Cholera*, pp.166-7.
32. *Glasgow Courier*, 13 March 1832; Thomas Shapter, *The History of the Cholera in Exeter in 1832*, London, 1849, reprint 1971, p.178; Minute Book of the Oxford Board of Health, 28 July 1832; Hugh Miller, *My Schools and Schoolmasters*, Edinburgh, 1878, p.488.
33. *Lancet*, 19 November 1831; Charles Taylor, *Partick – past and present*, Glasgow, 1902, p.79 (reference kindly given me by Mrs Sylvia Price of Edinburgh).
34. Thomas Brown, *A letter to the London Board of Health...on the pestilential cholera*, London, 1832, p.21.

35. *Cholera Gazette*, 14 January 1832.
36. *Fraser's Magazine*, vol.4, 1831, p.621; *Lancet*, 19 November 1831, p.281.
37. *Lancet*, vol.I, 1832, p.796.
38. *Reports on the Epidemic Cholera which raged throughout...India, since August 1819*, Government of Bombay, 1819, reported in *E.M.S.J.*, vol.16, 1820, p.458; Robert Venables, 'The nature and treatment of epidemic cholera', *London Medical and Physical Journal*, vol.58, 1832, p.416; *London Gazette*, 6 October 1848.
39. Harry Leake Gibbs, 'Observations on the Cholera', *E.M.S.J.*, vol.36, 1831, p.395; *Monthly Review*, vol.3, 1831, p.458; *Foreign Quarterly Review*, vol.8, 1831, p.473.
40. *E.M.S.J.*, vol.37, 1832, p.348; *John Bull*, 13 August 1832.
41. Thomas S. Kuhn, *The Structure of Scientific Revolutions*, 2nd edition, Chicago, 1970, and 'The function of dogma in scientific research' in A.C. Crombie (ed.), *Scientific Change*, London, 1963, reprinted in B. Barnes, *Sociology of Science*, London, 1972, pp.80-104; E.H. Ackerknecht, 'Anticontagionism between 1821 and 1867', *Bulletin of the History of Medicine*, vol.22, 1948, pp.562-93.
42. C. Bryce, 'An Examination of the Etiology of Cholera...', *Glasgow Medical Journal*, vol.5, 1832, p.272; *Lancet*, 19 November 1831, pp.259-63; E.M.S.J. vol.37, 1832, p.337; Henry Gaulter, *Malignant Cholera in Manchester*, p.26.
43. T. Oglier Ward, 'Observations upon the cholera as it appeared in Wolverhampton and neighbourhood', *Transactions of the Provincial Medical and Surgical Association*, vol.2, 1832, pp.368-90; James Eckford, *Facts and observations regarding the disease called epidemic cholera as it recently appeared in Prestonpans and its vicinity*, Edinburgh, 1832; *Lancet*, 19 November 1831 and 4 February 1832; *E.M.S.J.*, vol.37, 1832, pp.178-210.
44. Joseph Ayre, *A letter addressed to the Right Hon Lord Russell on the evil policy of quarantine...for arresting the progress of Asiatic cholera*, London, 1837; George Watt, *Glasgow Medical Journal*, vol.5, 1832; William Auchinlass, 'Report of the Epidemic Cholera as it visited the Town's Hospital, Glasgow in February and March 1832', *Glasgow Medical Journal*, vol.5, 1832. pp.113-18.
45. *E.M.S.J.*, vol.24, 1825, p.209; John Goss, *Practical Remarks on the disease called cholera which now exists on the continent of Europe*, London, 1831, p.20; John Lizars, *Investigations regarding Cholera Asphyxia...*, p.61.
46. *London Medical Gazette*, vol.9, 5 November 1831, p.163 and vol.10, 5 May 1832, p.165; *London Medical and Physical Journal*, vol.58, 1832, p.151.
47. *E.M.S.J.*, vol.28, 1828, p.424, review of Kennedy; *London Medical Gazette*, vol.9, 5 November 1831, p.163.
48. John Lizars, *Investigations regarding Cholera Asphyxia*, pp.20-5; James Kay dedicated his book on Manchester to the Scottish evangelical Thomas Chalmers.
49. William Bullock, *The History of Bacteriology*, London, 1938, pp.13-40; S.R. Bradbury, *The Evolution of the Microscope*, London, 1967, pp.108-235; *Lancet*, 19 November 1831, p.277; Adam Neale, *Linnaean Doctrine of Animate Contagions*, p.5 and 219.
50. John Lizars, *Investigations regarding Cholera Asphyxia*, pp.2-4 and 17-43; *Lancet*, 1832, *passim*; Post-Mortem Reports, P.R.O., P.C.1/103.
51. *E.M.S.J.*, vol.16, 1820, pp.566-71 and vol.17, 1821, pp.159-83 gives an excellent general account of the development of medical topography.
52. The studies referred to in the preceding paragraphs were, Rev. W. Leigh, *An authentic narrative of the melancholy occurrences at Bilston...during the awful visitation of cholera in that town...*, Wolverhampton, 1833; 'Cholera at Sedgley *Christian Observer*, vol.34, 1834, pp.1-17; Rev. Charles Girdleston, *Seven Sermons preached during the prevalence of the cholera in the parish of*

Sedgley, London, 1833; Rev. Vaughan-Thomas, *Memorials of the malignant cholera in Oxford, 1832*, Oxford, 1835; W. Haslewood and W. Mordey, *History and Medical Treatment of Cholera at Sunderland*, London, 1832; David Craigie, 'On the epidemic cholera of Newburn', *E.M.S.J.*, vol.37, 1832, pp.337-84; Thomas Proudfoot, 'Account of the Epidemic Cholera of Kendal', *E.M.S.J.*, vol.39, 1833, pp.70-103; Robert Baker, *Report to the Members of the Leeds Board of Health*, Leeds, 1833; Henry Gaulter, *The Origin and Progress of the Malignant Cholera in Manchester*, London, 1833. See also R.J. Morris, 'Religion and Medicine: The Cholera pamphlets of Oxford, 1832, 1849 and 1854', *Medical History*, vol.19, 1975, pp.256-70.
53. Whitelaw Ainslie, *Letters on Cholera*, pp.7-30, quoting Charles Wilkinson, *Elements of Galvanism*, 2 vols., London, 1804, vol.2, pp.288-9.
54. F.H. Garrison, *An introduction to the history of medicine*, 4th edition, Philadelphia, 1960, p.327; C.H. Wilkinson, *Elements of Galvanism*, vol.I, ch.2.
55. Adam Neale, *Linnaean Doctrine of Animate Contagions*, pp.215 and 237.
56. *The Monthly Review*, n.s., vol.3, 1831, p.450.

9 EPILOGUE

(i) The 'Lessons' of 1832

There was a wide-ranging, substantial and often violent reaction to the immediate impact of cholera. Long-term responses were not so clear. Men like Sir John Simon and Charles Creighton looked back at 1832 and saw obvious lessons in the epidemic. Cholera had demonstrated the relationship between disease and the dirty, ill-drained parts of towns and had shown the need for drainage, sewerage and filtered water supplies.[1] It ought to have been a spur to sanitary reform. Yet little action of this sort followed the epidemic.

1832 was one of those periodic occasions in the nineteenth century in which government and the middle classes made a shocked discovery of poverty. Charles Greville was alarmed by the information which came to him at the Privy Council, 'The awful thing is, the vast extent of misery and distress which prevails, and the evidence of the rotten foundations on which the whole fabric of this gorgeous society rests...'[2] Their Lordships were alarmed by what their agents found in Sunderland, '...these poor people have an undoubted right to a larger measure of relief than appears to have been dispensed.'[3] This reaction was in part an old pattern of social relationships; the aristocratic government intervening to ensure that the lower orders got their 'rights' from the middle classes. It also indicated the normal lack of contact between rulers and people. This gap was nearly as great at local level. Kay noticed it in Manchester. At Bilston, the middle class and their clergy expected to find some 500 families in extreme poverty, by which they meant needing relief at least twice a week. In fact they found 1,057 families in this position.[4]

In the winter of 1832-3, both government and people seemed to want to forget cholera as quickly as they could. The *Edinburgh Medical and Surgical Journal* declared they would review no more books on the subject because of 'the multitude of books which have recently issued from the press on the subject of cholera, and our determination no longer to try the patience of our readers'.[5] The newspaper and periodical Press dropped the subject even more rapidly than they had taken it up. Hence the work of James Kay, Gaulter and Robert Baker, which has received so much attention from historians, was largely ignored. The last letter in the Board of Health letter book showed that familiarity bred complacency:

> the disease will probably be contemplated henceforth in the same sanitary light as any other dangerous malady which may become domiciled in this country, its management must be left to the prudence and good feeling of those communities where it may occasionally show itself.[6]

Cholera played no part in social policy-making in the next decade. Although the discussion of poverty had a central place in the public and administrative reaction, the epidemic of 1832 had no place in the Poor Law Commission Report of 1834. Cholera did gain an occasional mention in the Commissioners' Local Reports to illustrate a point about surgeons' fees or to fill an item in the accounts, but the broader implications of the epidemic were ignored. The lessons of cholera had no place in the vast pamphlet literature which surrounded the Poor Law debate. Such lessons had no place in a 'reform' which was designed to reduce the amount of help which was given to the poor. Cholera had no place in the Factory Act debates. It had no mention in lesser debates, like the Select Committee on Drunkenness and the Select Committee on Public Walks, both published in 1833 and both on subjects which related to cholera as it was then understood.

There were two main reasons why the 'lessons' of cholera should have been ignored after 1832. First, the epidemic when it came was an anti-climax after the terrifying reading and speculation of 1831. British government had reacted to the approach of cholera with urgent attempts to find effective and responsible ways of stopping and treating the disease. Despite their failure these attempts were in marked contrast to the occasional pleading pamphlets which promoted smallpox vaccination. In part the initial reaction was prompted by fear of the unknown, in part by fear that the rich would be infected by the poor, though the belief that the rich would escape was equally powerful. The most important reason for taking such urgent action was the belief that cholera by its suddenness and unpredictability was capable of massive social and commercial disorganisation. Experience showed that this was not so in Britain. The unsatisfactory account which medicine gave of cholera supplied a second reason for lack of action. There were no clear 'lessons'. Certainly none which would justify increases in the rates. Indeed, the religious and moral accounts of cholera were more convincing to many and evoked more reaction.

Local evidence showed two sorts of long-term response to cholera

Epilogue

after 1832. The first was the Oxford pattern in which reforming energies were dissipated in activities which had little practical relationship to public health needs. The Oxford Board had noted the spread of cholera among the prostitutes of the New Hamel and resolved on a subscription to establish a charitable institution to help those women who wished to reform. Although the Board felt that they might take 'much higher and more comprehensive views of the subject', they closed their debate on the matter by 'entering upon the minutes the following propositions relating to the dangers to public health arising out of the profligacy, the destitution, the filthiness and the unwholesome situations of the residences of the common prostitute'.

It appears to this Board of great importance, viewing the matter in its lower instead of its higher affinities and entertaining it simply as a sanitary and precautionary measure that it would be conductive to public health and safety under the present calamity of cholerous sickness to effect some amelioration in the habits of the common prostitute — their homes and homesteads, the localities of their residences, their destitute as well as their debased condition, and generally in their natural and statistical as well as their spiritual and eternal relations.[7]

Although the Oxford Board saw the cholera among the prostitutes as part of the general prevalence of cholera in conditions of filth and poverty, the Board concerned themselves with that aspect of the New Hamel which attracted their attention on moral as well as public health grounds.

In Leeds the story was different. Here the strands of reform were created by the young Poor Law surgeon Robert Baker, and ran into the sands because of lack of public interest. He presented his report to the local Board of Health. It received a little notice in the local Press and council and was then forgotten.

The cholera of 1832 may be dismissed as an immediate influence on opinion regarding public health, but it was important for its influence on a number of individuals who later came to play key secondary roles in the public health campaigns after 1840. In 1839, Robert Baker returned to public notice with a statistical survey of the town which attracted a great deal of attention, which did not mention cholera, and which led to the 1842 Leeds Improvement Act. Reverend Charles Girdlestone, the Black Country parson of fervent evangelical views, took a leading part in religious and public health action against the cholera, and reappeared several years later as one of Chadwick's local informants for the 1842, *Report on the Sanitary Condition of the Labouring Population of Great Britain.* Baker was also amongst the local correspondents. In 1832 Duncan of Liverpool was given special thanks by the local board of health for his work. He was appointed as the first medical officer of health in 1847. James Kay's early experience of disease and poverty was gained among the cholera cases of south Manchester. He reappeared in the 1840s at the centre of work to improve the quality of schools and teachers among the working classes. There was then a sense in which a public health and a wider movement for the improvement of the conditions of the poor were created by the epidemic of 1832.

The powerful experience of observing and dealing with cholera came at the start of the careers of a small group of men. As these men were forming their impressions and evaluations of the society and environment in which they lived, they saw cholera, which through its pain and unpredictable spread emphasised the inhumanity and danger of British society. Ten or fifteen years later when they had gained in reputation, in social experience and authority, these people were able to influence the course of social and public health reform. If the lives of Baker, Duncan, Girdlestone and Kay prove to be characteristic of the lives of others, then the cholera of 1832 will be seen to have created the early cadres of a public health movement, which then went underground, to emerge again in the 1840s.[8]

(ii) **Cholera Returns**

When cholera returned in 1848 and 1849 there were many features of the epidemic which were familiar to those who had witnessed 1832. It visited the same places and found the same state of unpreparedness. Treatments and preventative measures all failed, and imperfect evidence suggests that the death rate was higher.

But there was a change in the dominant public mood which reflected greater changes in attitudes to health, government, religion and science,

> ...there is an improved condition of the public mind since 1832. The vague but intense alarm which preceded the former visitation of the epidemic, has been exchanged for a calm and rational view of the real amount of danger.[9]

After the epidemic there was none of the sudden loss of interest in cholera which had taken place in 1832. The *Edinburgh Review* and the

Christian Remembrancer both reviewed the government reports on the epidemic, whilst the medical journals showed none of the 'boredom' they had expressed in 1832. The *Edinburgh Medical and Surgical Journal,* the *Medical Times* and the *Lancet* continued to review books on cholera well into 1850, discussing new theories on its origin, printing letters on treatment as well as looking at the government publications.[10] There were several reasons for the change. During 1847, thousands of starving Irish people had fled from potato blight and brought typhus to the large cities of Britain. Those who had seen 'famine fever' in the crowded centres of Glasgow, Manchester and Leeds could not view cholera as an unprecedented horror.[11] The public health reports of the 1840s were slow to produce practical results in terms of government action, but through the many articles, pamphlets and public meetings they provoked, these reports gave public and government opinion a thorough education in science-based, especially miasma-based, attitudes to public health problems.[12]

Although they had little more to offer in 1849, the medical and scientific community were much more assured than they had been in 1832. Many doctors had seen cholera in 1832 and there were fewer disputes over the identity of the disease. The government was better informed. It had its own network of local agents, the local Registrars of Births, Deaths and Marriages, who were able to check reports by simple reference to death certificates. In addition, the General Board of Health employed two medical inspectors of their own, Drs Sutherland and Grainger, who were also able to check local reports and conditions. The new railway network meant they were able to do this with a speed impossible in 1832. The regular publication of weekly tables by the Registrar-General replaced the rumour and counter-rumour of the first epidemic. The profession itself was better organised for carrying out and discussing research. There was a network of journals which exchanged information across Europe. Most of the provincial hospitals had medical schools attached to them, and in the 1830s many towns had formed provincial medical societies which were a base for research. In addition the medical and scientific resources of London were greater, and included the increasing government interest in statistics.

There was the same confusion over treatment. The most important change was one of emphasis. The profession had 'discovered' in 1832 that nearly all cases of cholera were preceded by premonitory diarrhoea.[13] Searle explained the logic of this. Cholera, dysentery, diarrhoea and typhoid all had the same basic cause and were modifications of each other. It was natural that under certain conditions one form of the disease would develop from another. Many thousands of cases of diarrhoea were treated through house-to-house visitations, upon which boards of health confidently congratulated themselves that they had prevented many cases of cholera. Novelties were tried. Chloroform used by Simpson in Edinburgh as a pain-killer during childbirth was tried. A bed with anti-static legs was proposed to counter electrical influences. There was a dim memory but little interest in Latta's method, and Dr George Johnson, physician at King's College Hospital, achieved some notoriety by his 'eliminative' treatment in which he assisted the natural course of cholera with huge doses of castor oil.[14]

The real sign of assurance came over etiology. The old contagionists still held their views, but miasmatic thinking dominated official medical and government statements. When the Royal College of Physicians asked for the views of members they had 84 replies: 32 rejected contagion and only 7 gave unqualified support. The others were uncertain or held that both modes of diffusion could operate under different conditions. The recently created General Board of Health, like its secretary Edwin Chadwick, was aggressively miasmatic.[15] The ready acceptance of this theory was helped not only by the public health campaigns of the 1840s but also by the methodology of an increasing number of statistical studies of disease. These depended on figures gathered by geographical area. Hence attention was directed to localised influences which in turn, with the help of the nauseating smell of many of these areas, was related to miasma.

It is tempting to attribute the dominance of miasmatic thought to the increasing influence of the middle class. Whilst this paradigm had gained influence through middle-class groups and research sponsored by commercial interests, it now had a logic of its own, which gave the paradigm an authority with all manner of governments and social groups quite independent of class or sectional interest. By 1848, miasma had been accepted by autocratic Russia as well as bourgeois Britain.[16]

By contrast, whether as cause or effect, the religious response was more muted. There was no official day of fasting, prayer and humiliation, though many churches appointed their own individual day. Such rituals had by no means been rejected. A few months after the 1854 epidemic, the nation went to prayer for success in the Crimea. The God of cholera had become the God of battles. Hugh Miller in his Free Church paper the *Witness* saw the ritual with almost anthropological clarity. It was unwise, he said, to rely on 'natural laws' alone. 'Society is a moral being and demands something more'.

Epilogue

> A whole people prostrate at the footstool of the Supreme, owning their sins and acknowledging that they have received merited chastisement, yet casting themselves upon the clemency and grace of the Majesty they have offended...Nor will such an act be unproductive of the happiest results for society itself.

These acts of worship confirmed the values and unity of the community. Indeed, the very existence of that community depended upon the acknowledgement of their collective awareness of God. The day of prayer was 'an outward and visible sign' of their relationship to God's moral government. 'It tends to conserve order and good government.'[17]

God the Avenger was not dead but in retreat. He survived among the Wesleyan Methodists who had their only cholera revival at Redruth in Cornwall. Christ the Mediator played a more important part. Sentimentality replaced savagery,

> ...only one in our circle has been thus removed as yet; and of her eternal gain, by death, no-one who knew her has even the shadow of a doubt. Her class in the Sunday Schools cannot think of heaven now without thinking of her. Oh, copy, so far as you are teachers her lovely example and sweet spirit.[18]

All denominations, and even the evangelicals were much less confident and clear about the relationship between sin and cholera. Drink still had a central place in such thinking. The epidemic was obviously another call to prayer. But the sins of the individual were being replaced by sins of omission on the part of the nation. By 1848 Providence and public health went very nicely together. As the United Presbyterians said in Scotland,

> there is reason to hope that, under the blessing of God, attention to sanitary regulations issued by the national Board of Health will prove effectual in mitigating greatly if not in arresting this awful judgement.[19]

The Bishop of London represented the change in religious mood as neatly as any one individual. In 1832, he had taken care to place Providence in both Cholera Acts. In the intervening years he had come to see material poverty as a major barrier between the Church and the working classes and had given special attention to housing and sanitation. In November 1849 he preached in St Paul's. He began with Providence and the Psalms, with Nineveh, the destroying angel, reaping in the whirlwind and chastising the sinner for his worldliness. God the legitimator was called on as guardian of the social order. The epidemic was 'the surest antidote to the poison of infidelity, disloyalty and anarchy...let us endeavour to show our thankfulness by supplying the people with increased means of education and public worship'. He went on in a new mood, that of God the reformer,

> The most suitable and I believe the most acceptable mode of acknowledging the goodness of God in withdrawing the scourge of pestilence, and preserving to us the kindly fruits of the earth, will be by a larger measure of charitable consideration for the physical evils which affect our poorer brethren...Want of decent cleanly habitations is one of the chief evils that affect the poor...At present neatness order and comfort are unknown in their miserable overcrowded dwellings; modesty is impracticable, delicacy of feeling destroyed, and coarseness of language and manners prevail, and prepare the mind for vicious intercourse in future years. None of the comforts of home are there — none of its softening purifying influences; and can we wonder if in such sinks of immorality, if spared by disease, the scandals and pests of society, the mendicant, the drunkard and the thief are produced?[20]

This change in religious mood took place before medical science had produced any convincing account of cholera. The God of cholera represented the social and metaphysical attitudes of those who were dominant in forming the religious consciousness of Britain, and was not primarily a God of the gaps.

(iii) The Public Health Acts of 1848

As cholera approached Britain in the summer of 1848, two important public health acts were passed through Parliament, the Public Health Act itself and the Nuisance Removal and Contagious Diseases Act. The first created a General Board of Health with powers to initiate and assist local sanitary reform projects. The second gave the General Board power to issue orders and instructions, but only on the authority and after an order from the Privy Council. The passage of these Acts was often linked to fears of the approaching cholera. The debates in Parliament do not suggest that the link was important. True, when the Commons were considering amendments from the Lords, Morpeth treated them to a reading of the cholera death toll from Russia, but it was unlikely that

Epilogue 205

this convinced anyone not already attracted to the Bill. Some even suggested that cholera was too dangerous to be tackled through such a complex and contentious measure, and suggested that the simpler 1832 Act was more appropriate. When Morpeth introduced the Bill in February 1848, he told the House,

> I do not wish to lay any material stress upon the possible approach of cholera...it is far from any temporary evil, any transient visitation against which our legislation is now called upon to provide. It is the abiding host of disease, the endemic not the epidemic pestilence, the permanent overhanging mist of infection, the slaughter doubling its ravages on our bloodiest fields of conflict, that we are now summoned to grapple with.

If the 1848 Acts can be attributed to any one disease, that disease must be typhus, for it was the one most frequently mentioned in the debates and in the decade of parliamentary reports which preceded the two Acts. The approach of cholera did not prevent the House of Commons using all possible means to delay the Bill and stripping the General Board of all its major powers in the name of protecting the localities from central power. The fear of cholera had a marginal effect in reducing delays in late summer 1848. The Bishop of London withdrew amendments in the Lords designed to strengthen the Bill because he felt that delay in the face of cholera was irresponsible. Thus the approach of cholera weakened the Bill because it rushed the health reformers without forcing the hand of anti-centralisers like Colonel Sibthorpe. Fear of cholera did nothing to hurry the government into producing measures which filled the gaps in public health legislation left by the Act — in the introduction of measures for London, for Scotland, or for the prohibition of interment in overcrowded city graveyards. The real cholera act of 1848 was the Nuisance Removal and Disease Prevention Act which went through with commendable dispatch largely because its major principles had been agreed during the passage of a temporary Act the previous year.[21]

Throughout 1849, the administrative burden of cholera was met by the General Board of Health. The Board, created by the 1848 Act, consisted of a Minister, Viscount Morpeth, an unpaid member, Lord Ashley and a paid member, Edwin Chadwick. The last two together with their two medical inspectors, Grainger and Sutherland, did most of the work during the epidemic.[22] They were active, powerless, derided and largely ineffective. The Public Health Act itself was of little value to them — the intended gains of this Act were long-term, setting up local boards of health with plans for drainage, sewerage and water supply. The General Board was constituted on 22 September, a few days before the first cases of cholera were announced. 'We have indeed toiled unceasingly, and not as mere officials but with earnestness and feeling', wrote Ashley at the end of the epidemic, but earnestness and good feeling were not enough.[23] They issued instructions and regulations and sent their medical inspectors into the field, but found that the temporary powers granted to them by the Privy Council under the Diseases Prevention Act enabled them to help the willing but not to coerce the unwilling. In Sheffield, cleansing and early medical aid was thorough and deaths were reduced to 46. Dumfries needed a visit from Dr Sutherland before action was taken, but the London parishes were made of sterner stuff and resisted all attempts to persuade them to take extra measures until the middle of September when some of the worst hit began house-to-house visitation.[24] The General Board got little help and attention from leading members of the governing classes. Whilst cholera spread in London, the Queen was in the Highlands, the Prime Minister deerstalking and the Archbishop relaxing in the Lake District. In many ways the structure of local government was less appropriate than it had been in 1832. Then *ad hoc* committees had been formed and, once endowed with power, had acted quite well within the limitations of their knowledge. In 1848 and 1849 the task was given to the local Boards of Guardians whose natural habits were to restrict spending and then limit it to relief rather than preventive measures.[25] Despite the cleansing and house-to-house visitations which the General Board felt had saved many lives, it was probably more ineffective in its own terms than the Central Board had been, and equally ineffective in real terms.

(iv) The Partial Solution

The summer of 1849 marked the high noon of miasmatic theory. By the end of the year confidence in the theory had been weakened by its failure, and by the scientific work of John Snow, and a group of doctors in Bristol.

The work of Budd, Swayne and Brittain in Bristol was made possible by the improvement of the microscope and by the development of the provincial medical societies. Bristol had an active medical community centred on its general hospital, the medical school and the Bristol Medico-Chirugical Society, which set up a sub-committee '...for the microscopic investigation of choleraic evacuations'. In the course of this research Swayne and Brittain found distinctive annular bodies which

Epilogue

grew progressively in size. Specimens were sent to Quekett at the Royal College of Surgeons who agreed that they were 'of a fungoid nature'. William Budd, a leading local physician already known for his work on typhus and typhoid, was prepared to take his inferences much further than the other two men. He found the same objects in the drinking water of places infected with cholera, and concluded that the cause of cholera was 'a living organism of a distinct species, which was taken by the act of swallowing it, which multiplied in the intestine by self propagation. . .' The disruption thus caused derived from the 'enormous chemical power which plants possess to supply themselves with material for their growth'. Baly and Gull, the leading members of the Cholera Committee of the Royal College of Physicians, immediately investigated these claims but found that the particles described were not always present in cholera-infected water, and identified them as partially digested food. The rapid rise and fall of the fungus theory of the origin of cholera showed how well-organised the medical community had become since 1832. The theory was immediately published and immediate notice was taken by the London leadership of the profession. These empirically tested and logically consistent predictions were subjected to mutual evaluation and in this case found wanting, not for reasons of prestige or social pressure but by those same scientific rules of observation and logic.[26] The fall of the fungus theory was unfortunate for it discredited other 'water-borne' theories like that of John Snow, but the investigations had shown that particles from intestines could turn up in drinking water. There were now good scientific reasons for suspecting sewage-tainted water apart from the smell. The 1850s saw a sustained parliamentary campaign to improve the water supply of London which brought slow results.[27]

Of the two routes to the understanding of cholera which had been blocked in 1832, the Bristol men had chosen microscopic studies. John Snow linked his prestige as an influential London surgeon to the analytical power of descriptive statistics. The early papers he wrote in 1853 showed that his inferences had begun with observations on the pathology and clinical history of the disease in the traditional manner. Cholera, he wrote, 'always commences with disturbances of the functions of the alimentary canal; all the early symptoms are connected with this canal, and the effects which follow are only the results of what have occurred.'[28] Thus he looked for some poison, which he believed came from the excreta of cholera patients and was swallowed by the new victims. His attention was drawn to a number of instances in which water supplies polluted with sewage had been the common factor in an explosive outbreak of cholera. He was especially impressed by the deaths in middle-class Albion Terrace in Wandsworth where a stockbroker and a surgeon's daughter had been amongst those who had died after the overflow pipe from a sewer had poured water into the water supply system from a nearby spring.[29] When Snow published the first edition of *On the mode of communication of cholera* it aroused considerable interest, but few were convinced by this rather slight volume of scattered examples which illustrated, as events subsequently proved, a brilliant intuition. Snow admitted that the evidence was imperfect but he published so that he might lay claim to that prestige which science grants to those who first publish an original and successful idea.

When cholera returned to London in 1854 Snow was ready. Events presented him with two massive experiments which demonstrated his theory with convincing clarity. He directed his attention to the districts of Kennington, Waterloo, Lambeth, St George Southwark and St Peter Walworth which were supplied by the Vauxhall Water Company which drew water from the sewage-laden Thames at Battersea Fields, and by the Lambeth Company, which had been one of the first to respond to the pressure for purer supplies, and drew water from a new position at Thames Ditton.

> No fewer than three hundred thousand people of both sexes, of every age and occupation, and of every rank and station from gentlefolks down to the very poor, were divided into two groups without their choice, and, in most cases without their knowledge; one group being supplied with water containing the sewage of London and, amongst it, whatever might have come from the cholera patients, and the other group having water quite free from such impurity.[30]

The cholera cases he identified through information given him by the Registrar-General. The water company of the victim he identified by a silver nitrate test which showed up the high quantity of common salt in the Vauxhall Company product. As Snow said coolly, it was 'part of that which has passed through the kidneys and bowels of two millions and a quarter of the inhabitants of London'.[31] The results of the experiment were striking (Table 13, p.209).

If this were not enough he had his Broad Street experience to quote. He had investigated an explosive outbreak in this area of Soho and found that the Broad Street pump was a factor common to most cases.

Table 13: Cholera Deaths and Water Supplies in London[32]

	Pop. 1851	Cholera deaths in 14 weeks ending 14 Oct	Deaths per 10,000 living
Houses supplied by Southwark and Vauxhall	266,516	4,093	153
Houses supplied by Lambeth Co.	173,748	461	26

He persuaded the parish authorities to remove the handle of the pump and the epidemic faded. It was only with the help of the church that he found the source of infection. Rev. Henry Whitehead, curate of St Luke's, had recently graduated from Oxford and was one of an increasing number of clergy who sought to serve God by social reform as well as saving souls. He knew the affairs of the parish better than any visiting surgeon and found that just before the epidemic a child had died in No.40 Broad Street from exhaustion following diarrhoea, but that the symptoms were those of cholera. The child's nappies had been steeped and the water thrown down a sink and into a cesspool which seeped into the pump well.[33] The second edition was a convincing and compelling statement of his case. Snow realised that the argument still had its social and political dimension and assured his readers that accepting the water-borne theory of cholera implied prevention by 'simple measures that will not interfere with social and commercial intercourse'. Snow had reconciled the needs of industrial *laissez-faire* society with contagionist theory.[34]

The immediate impact of Snow's theory has disappointed many historians who find that he made no sweeping conversion of the profession and received little mention in medical textbooks or subsequent works on cholera. In 1854, the Scientific Committee of the re-formed General Board of Health attacked the theory at its weakest point. Neither Snow nor the committee could-identify the nature of the 'cholera poison' in the water. This had to wait for the work of Robert Koch in Alexandria in 1883.[35] Snow's impact was greater than this neglect and criticism suggests. He was careful to present his theory as a partial solution. Water was not the only means by which cholera was transmitted. He also linked his inferences to the prestigious activities of pathology and collecting case histories. Men like John Simon, medical officer of the City of London, rejected the theory at the start but by 1856 he was publishing, unacknowledged, very similar views. Thomas Acland, leader of the medical profession in Oxford, wrote a powerful miasmatic account of the 1854 epidemic there, but the measures he adopted included shutting off the water supply of the prison, a policy straight from Snow. In 1849, Acland had done no more than recommend an improved diet for the prison.[36] Snow's real triumph came in 1866 after his death. William Farr at the Registrar-General's office had been convinced by Snow's theory; 'I was thus prepared in 1866 to closely scrutinize the water supply.' When an explosive epidemic hit East London in July he did just this, and, despite the denials of company officials he rapidly traced the source of the epidemic to the Old Ford works of the East London Water Company, where open ponds of water tainted by sewage from the nearby River Lea were being used as an emergency reserve of water by the Company. As soon as this practice was stopped, the epidemic died.[37]

This was the last of the great 'experiments' from which the Registrar-General's office gathered data which demonstrated Snow's theory. Cholera was defeated in a grim game of scientific inference and political resistance. British society finally outwitted the cholera with a technology of sewers, water pipes and artesian wells, a network of information with the Registrar-General at its centre, and an administration almost as confused, overlapping and ill-co-ordinated as it had been in 1832, but a little less powerless. Cholera had been blindly admitted to Britain in 1832. The men who curbed its spread in 1866 were a little less blind though their understanding was by no means complete. God the scientist emerged slowly from the mists of miasma and the fires of vengeance which had obscured the workings of natural law in 1832.

Notes

1. Charles Creighton, *A history of epidemics in Great Britain*, 2 vols., Cambridge, 1891-4, vol.2, pp.793-862; Sir John Simon, *English Sanitary Institutions*, London, 1890.
2. *The Greville Memoirs...*, vol.II, pp.214 and 284.
3. Central Board of Health Letter Book, 22 November 1831, P.R.O., P.C.1/93.
4. *Wesleyan Methodist Magazine*, vol.55, 1832, p.203.
5. *The Greville Memoirs...*, vol.II, p.284; *E.M.S.J.*, vol.40, 1833, p.177.
6. Central Board of Health Letter Book, 15 August 1833, P.R.O., P.C.1/93.
7. Oxford Board of Health Minute Book, 9 September 1832.
8. W.R. Lee, 'Robert Baker: The First Doctor in the Factory Department', *British Journal of Industrial Medicine*, vol.21, 1964, pp.85-93; Rev. Charles Girdlestone, *Seven Sermons preached during the prevalence of cholera in the parish of Sedgley*, London, 1833; 'The Cholera at Sedgley', *The Christian Observer*, vol.34, 1834, pp.1-16; Frank Smith, *The Life of Sir James*

Epilogue 211

Kay-Shuttleworth, London, 1923; W.M. Frazer, *Duncan of Liverpool*, London, 1947, p.49; Edwin Chadwick, *Report on the Sanitary Condition of the Labouring Population of Great Britain*, 1842, edited by M.W. Flinn.
9. *Monthly Journal of Medical Science*, vol.9, 1848, p.349.
10. *The Christian Remembrancer*, vol.19, 1850, pp.164-85 reviewed the *Quarterly Returns...of the Registrar-General* and the *Edinburgh Review*, vol.96, 1852, pp.403-35 looked at the *Report of the General Board of Health on the Epidemic Cholera of 1848 and 1849*.
11. *Free Church Magazine*, vol.5, 1848, p.367; *The People's Journal*, vol.4, p.344; Cecil Woodham Smith, *The Great Hunger*, London, pp.266-81.
12. *Edinburgh Review*, vol.96, 1852, pp.403-35; M.W. Flinn, Introduction to the Chadwick Report..., pp.66-73.
13. *Report on the Cholera epidemic of 1866 in England*, supplement to the 29th annual report of the Registrar-General..., P.P.(H. of C.) 1867-8, vol.37; *Medical Times*, 25 December 1847.
14. *Medical Times*, 11 August, 9 September and 14 October 1848, and 20 January, 23 June and 22 September 1849; *Monthly Journal of Medical Science*, vol.8, 1849, p.393; *Once a Week*, vol.2, 1868, pp.33-6; *Contemporary Review*, vol.10, 1869, pp.114-21.
15. *E.M.S.J.*, vol.72, 1849, p.201; *Monthly Journal of Medical Science*, vol.9, 1848, p.349; *Medical Times*, 16 October 1847; W. Bailey and W. Gull, *Reports on the Epidemic Cholera drawn up at the desire of the Cholera Committee of the Royal College of Physicians*, London, 1854, pp.3-4.
16. E.H. Ackerknecht, 'Anti-contagionism between 1821 and 1867', *Bulletin of the History of Medicine*, vol.22, 1948, p.580.
17. *The Witness*, 25 August 1849; Hugh Miller, *My Schools and Schoolmasters*, Edinburgh, 1878, p.554.
18. *Christian Witness*, 1849, p.480.
19. *The United Presbyterian Magazine*, vol.2, 1848, p.528.
20. Rev. George Biber, *Bishop Bloemfield and his times*, London, 1857, pp.77-88, 124-41; Alfred Bloemfield, *A Memoir of Charles James Bloemfield, D.D.*, 2 vols., London, 1863, vol.I, p.177 and vol.II, p.113; *A pastoral letter to the clergy of the Diocese of London*, by Charles James, Bishop of London, London, 1847; *Illustrated London News*, 17 November 1849.
21. The major debates took place between 10 February and 31 August 1848, when both Bills received the Royal Assent, *Hansard's Parliamentary Debates*, 3rd series, vol.96 to vol.101, 1848. See also *People's Journal*, vol.6, 1848, p.213; *Tait's Edinburgh Magazine*, n.s., vol.16, 1849, pp.121-2.
22. R. Lambert, *Sir John Simon and English Social Administration*, London, 1963, p.71; Edwin Hodder, *The life and work of the Seventh Earl of Shaftesbury*, London, 1887, p.417.
23. Hodder, *Seventh Earl of Shaftesbury*, p.418.
24. *Report of the General Board of Health on the epidemic Cholera of 1848 and 1849*, appendix A, pp.47-59, and 107-11, Appendix B, pp.130-45, P.P.(H. of C.) 1850, vol.21; 'Seventh Notification with reference to the measures of prevention and relief of cholera adopted in the Metropolis, 18 September 1849', *London Gazette*, 1849, p.2,859; *Times*, 26 September 1849.
25. 1849 *Report...*, p.137; 'Seventh Notification...', p.2,863; *Medical Times*, 23 December 1848.
26. Evidence for the fungous origin of cholera, *E.M.S.J.*, vol.73, 1850, pp.81-118; William Budd, *Malignant Cholera: its mode of propagation*, London, 1849; E.W. Goodall, *William Budd*, Bristol, 1936.
27. *Edinburgh Medical Journal*, vol.82, 1855, pp.93-4; *Medical Times*, 29 October 1853.

28. *Medical Times*, 1 October 1853.
29. John Snow, *On the Mode of Communication of Cholera*, 1st edition, London, 1849; *Times*, 9 August 1849; Wade Hampton Frost, 'Introduction to John Snow', *On the Mode of Communication of Cholera*, reprint of the 2nd edition, New York, 1936.
30. John Snow, *Communication of Cholera*, 2nd edition, p.75.
31. *Medical Times*, 30 September 1854.
32. John Snow, *Communication of Cholera*, 2nd edition, p.88.
33. *Medical Times*, 23 September 1854; John Snow, *Communication of Cholera*, pp.39-54; *Report on the Cholera outbreak in the parish of St James, Westminster during the autumn of 1854*, presented to the vestry by the Cholera Inquiry Committee, July 1855, London, 1855; Rev. H.D. Rawnsley, *Henry Whitehead, 1825-1896*, Glasgow, 1898, pp.29-42 and 206; G. Kitson Clark, *Churchmen and the condition of England*, London, 1973.
34. John Snow, *Communication of Cholera*, 1st edition, p.30.
35. *Report of the Committee for Scientific Enquiries in relation to the Cholera Epidemic of 1854: General Board of Health (Medical Council)*. P.P.(H. of C.), 1854-5, vol.21; A.H. Abou-Gareeb, 'Koch's contribution to cholera', *Journal of the Indian Medical Association*, vol.46, 1966, pp.543-9.
36. *Journal of Public Health*, vol.2, 1856, p.192; R. Lambert, *Sir John Simon*, p.51; H.W. Acland, *Memoir of the Cholera at Oxford in the year 1854*, Oxford, 1856, p.46.
37. *Report on the Cholera epidemic of 1866. . .; Medical Times and Gazette*, 8 September 1866.

10 REFLECTIONS

Shuddering humanity asks, 'Who are these?
And what their crime?' – *They fell by one disease!*
By the blue pest, whose grip no art can shun,
No force unwrench, out-singled one by one;
When, like a monstrous birth, the womb of fate
Bore a new death of unrecorded date,
And doubtful name. – Far east the fiend begun
Its course; thence round the world pursued the sun,
The ghosts of millions followed at its back,
Whose desecrated graves betrayed their track.
On Albion's shores unseen the invader step;
Secret and swift through field and city sweep;
At noon, at midnight, seized the weak, the strong,
Asleep, awake, alone, amid the throng;
Kill'd like a murderer; fix'd its icy hold,
And rung out life with agony of cold;
Nor stay's its vengeance where it crush'd the prey,
But set a mark like Cain's upon their clay,
And this tremendous seal impress'd on all, –
'Bury me out of sight and out of call.'

When James Montgomery stood in the cholera burial ground in Sheffield and wrote these lines he was not perhaps stirred to great poetry, but he expressed the sense of awe, terror and guilt which cholera aroused.[1]

It was this power of cholera to evoke such strong feeling that made it such a harsh test of British society. As a test it indicated the underlying stability of that society in 1832. There was a swift reaction to discontent, which brought a rapid return to equilibrium in relationships which aroused much bitterness.

The year 1832 also revealed the importance of moral and metaphysical assumptions in the response to disease. This must be given more importance in the history of public health. The energies devoted to prayer and fasting were not a mark of fatalism but of patterns of thought which are even now only partly rejected. Similar problems still survive with many aspects of mental illness. Medical treatment or a loud cry of 'pull yourself together' may greet those who announce they are depressed depending on whether they place their statement in the context of moral or clinical assumptions. When mental illness and violence are mixed, the problem of separating moral punishment from scientific treatment is as difficult as it was for the Methodist who stood on Bottle Bank in Christmas week 1831. Moral and religious assumptions about disease never came to an end in Britain, but they were dismissed from their place in official thinking by Lord Palmerston in his famous reply to the Presbytery of Edinburgh who had asked him to declare a national fast day in 1854,

> Lord Palmerston would suggest, that the best course which the people of this country can pursue to deserve that the further progress of the cholera should be stayed, will be to employ the interval that will elapse between the present time and the beginning of next spring, in planning and executing measures by which those portions of their towns and cities which are inhabited by the poorest classes, and which, from the nature of things, must most need purification and improvement, may be freed from those causes and sources of contagion, which, if allowed to remain, will infallibly breed pestilence and be fruitful in death, in spite of all the prayers and fastings of a united but inactive nation. When man has done his utmost for his own safety, then is the time to invoke the blessing of heaven to give effect to his exertions.[2]

This was regarded as good sense but bad theology. The government had recognised that health was a secular matter.

Cholera revealed the social pressures on the development of science, and the manner in which the incomplete and uncertain logic of scientific argument increased the vulnerability of the scientific world to outside pressures. There were the internal pressures of the scientific community which still exist, pressures produced by the distribution of research resources and publication opportunity, pressures felt by Thomas Latta, pressures of prestige upon innovation. It was rare for a man to choose his theory solely to suit his own economic or class interest, or to please his patients and paymasters. This process was more subtle than this. Prestige, influence, space in periodicals naturally went to those whose views were compatible with the needs of the powerful and wealthy, whether among the medical, commercial or aristocratic élites. John Snow, who had argued against prevailing opinion for several years, understood the process well.

Reflections 215

The great injury which strict quarantine would do this nation, and the ruin it would entail to particular interests, was a great obstacle to the general admission that cholera was a communicable disease. He did not mean that individuals knowingly shaped their opinions for these reasons, but that they were unconsciously influenced by them.[3]

His friend William Farr as a civil servant saw a different aspect of the influence of economic interest on scientific opinion,

....in recent times air has had its sectaries, and so has water; but as the air of London is not supplied like water by companies, the air had the worst of it, both before parliamentary committees and Royal Commissions. For air no scientific witnesses have been retained, no learned counsel have pleaded...[4]

Social and economic pressures may still influence science in the choice of research projects or in the selections of different aspects of a discovery for development, but the greater completeness of scientific logic makes it less likely that sectional and class interests can line up behind competing schools of thought. Economics is still in its pre-scientific phase. British economic policy since 1950 has been a long drawn-out agony based on even greater theoretical confusions than the cholera men of 1832 experienced. Theories of wage push, cost push and monetary inflation attract supporters who have a keen eye on the impact which the policy implication of each theory will have on the interest which they represent. No one has yet done for economics what germ theory did for medicine.

The historian of cholera gains access to the past through the pain and fear of many thousands of people. The reality of their experience has survived in registers, letters, periodicals, minute books and newspapers,

> That the past experience revived in the meaning
> Is not the experience of one life only
> But of many generations — not forgetting
> Something that is probably quite ineffable:
> The backward look behind the assurance
> Of recorded history, the backward half look
> Over the shoulder, towards the primitive terror.
> Now we come to discover that the moments of agony

(Whether, or not, due to misunderstanding,
Having hoped for the wrong things or dreaded the wrong things
Is not in question) are likewise permanent
With such permanence as time has. We appreciate this better
In the agony of others, nearly experienced,
Involving ourselves, than in our own.
For our own past is covered by the currents of action,
But the torment of others remains an experience
Unqualified, unworn by subsequent attrition.
People change, and smile: but the agony abides,
Time the destroyer is time the preserver.[5]

Notes

1. *The Poetical Works of James Montgomery,* collected by himself, London, 1851, p.338.
2. Edwin Hodder, *The life and work of the Seventh Earl of Shaftesbury,* London, 1887, p.485.
3. *Medical Times,* 16 January 1858.
4. *Report on the Cholera Epidemic of 1866...,* P.P.(H. of C.), 1867-8, vol.37, p.lxxix.
5. T.S. Eliot, 'The Dry Salvages', from *The Four Quartets,* London, 1944.

SELECT BIBLIOGRAPHY

Public Record Office, London

Papers of the Central Board of Health, P.C.1/93 to 105

British Parliamentary Papers

Copies of extracts of all information communicated to His Majesty's Government relative to the Cholera Morbus, 1831, vol.18

Report of the General Board of Health on the epidemic cholera in 1848-49, 1850, vol.21

Report of the committee for Scientific Enquiries in relation to the cholera epidemic of 1854: General Board of Health, 1854-55, vol.21

Report on the cholera epidemic of 1866, supplement to the 29th annual report of the Registrar-General for Births, Deaths and Marriages, 1867-68, vol.37

Newspapers and Periodicals Consulted

Asiatic Journal
British Critic (orthodox Church of England)
Carpenter's Monthly Political Magazine
Catholic Magazine and Review, Birmingham
Cholera Gazette, January 1832 to April 1832
Christian Observer (evangelical church of England)
Cobbett's Political Register
Congregational Magazine
The Courier
The Covenanter, Belfast and Glasgow (extreme Presbyterian)
Eclectic Review
Edinburgh Evening Courant
Edinburgh Medical and Surgical Journal, 1817-1850
Evangelical Magazine
Foreign Quarterly Review
Fraser's Magazine
Glasgow Medical Magazine
John Bull
Lancet
London Gazette

London Medical Gazette
London Medical and Physical Journal, 1818-1833
Loyal Reformer's Gazette, Glasgow
Missionary Register (evangelical clergy and Anglican missionary societies)
The Monthly Repository (Unitarian)
The Monthly Review
New Monthly Magazine
The Phrenological Journal
Poor Man's Advocate (edited by John Doherty), Manchester
Poor Man's Guardian (edited by Henry Hetherington), London
The Times, London
United Services Magazine
Wesleyan Methodist Magazine
Westminster Review

Contemporary Publications

H.W. Acland, *Memoir on the cholera at Oxford in the year 1854, with considerations suggested by the epidemic*, London, 1856

W.F. Ainsworth, *Observations on pestilential cholera at Sunderland*, London, 1832

J. Alderson, *A brief outline of the history and progress of the cholera in Hull*, London, 1832

H.K. Armstrong and S. Edgar, *Observations on malignant cholera...at Prestonpans, Cockenzie and Port Seton...*, Edinburgh, 1832

J.B. Atlay, Sir Henry Wentworth Acland, London, 1903

W. Bailey and W. Gull, *Reports on the epidemic cholera drawn up at the desire of the Royal College of Physicians*, London, 1854

Robert Baker, *Report to the members of the Leeds Board of Health*, Leeds, 1833

George Hamilton Bell, *Treatis on cholera asphyxia*, Edinburgh, 1831

George Hamilton Bell, *Letter to Sir Henry Halford on the tendency of the proposed regulations...*, Edinburgh, 1831

William Budd, *Malignant cholera, its mode of propagation and prevention*, London, 1849

T.W. Chevalier, *On Asiatic cholera*, London, 1831

Alexander Turnbull Christie, *A treatis on the epidemic cholera*, London, 1833

W. Reid Clanny, *Hyperanthraxis; or the cholera at Sunderland*, London, 1832

Henry Cooper, 'On the cholera mortality in Hull during the

the epidemic of 1849', *Journal of the Statistical Society of London*, 1853

Directions to plain people as a guide for their conduct in the cholera, London, 1831

William Farr, 'The influence of elevation on the fatality of cholera', *Journal of the Statistical Society of London*, 1853

Henry Gaulter, *The origins and progress of the malignant cholera in Manchester*, Manchester, 1833

G. Girdlestone, *Seven sermons preached during the prevalence of cholera in the parish of Sedgley*, London, 1833

John Goss, *Practical remarks on the disease called cholera which now exists on the continent of Europe*, London, 1831

W. Haslewood and W. Mordey, *History and medical treatment of cholera at Sunderland*, London, 1832

Bissett Hawkins, *History of the epidemic spasmodic cholera of Russia*, London, 1831

James P. Kay, *The moral and physical condition of the working classes employed in the cotton manufacture of Manchester*, Manchester, 1832

James Butler Kell, *Cholera at Sunderland in 1831*, Edinburgh, 1834

James Kennedy, *The history of the contagious cholera with facts explanatory of its origin and laws, and of a rational method of cure*, London, 1831

William Leigh, *An authentic narrative of the melancholy occurrences at Bilston... during the awful visitation of the town by cholera*, Wolverhampton, 1833

A.C. MacLaren, 'On the origin and spread of cholera in the 8th district of Plympton St Mary Devonshire', *Journal of the Statistical Society of London*, 1850

William MacMichael, *Is the cholera spasmodica of India a contagious disease...a letter addressed to Sir Henry Halford*, London, 1831

Adam Neale, *Researches to establish the truth of the Linnaean doctrine of animate contagion*, London, 1832

J.P. Needham, *Facts and observations relative to cholera as it prevailed in the City of York*, London, 1832

Charles Searle, *Cholera, its nature, causes and treatment*, London, 1830

Thomas Shapter, *The history of cholera in Exeter in 1832*, London, 1849

John Snow, *On the mode of communication of cholera*, first edition, London, 1849, second edition enlarged, London, 1855, reprinted with introduction by Wade Hampton Frost, New York, 1936

220 Select Bibliography

Charles Turner Thackrah, *Cholera, its character and treatment...with reference to the disease as now existing in Newcastle and neighbourhood*, London, 1832

Rev. Vaughan Thomas, *Memorials of the malignant cholera in Oxford 1832*, Oxford, 1835

Secondary Literature

E.H. Ackernecht, 'Anti-contagionism between 1821 and 1867', *Bulletin of the History of Medicine*, vol.22, 1948

E. Ashworth Underwood, 'The history of cholera in Great Britain', *Proceedings of the Royal Society of Medicine*, vol.41, 1948

———, 'The history of the 1832 cholera epidemic in Yorkshire', *Proceedings of the Royal Society of Medicine*, vol.28, 1935

———, 'The cholera epidemic in Exeter 1832', *British Medical Journal*, 1933

George W. Baker and Dwight D. Chapman (eds.), *Man and Society in Disaster*, New York, 1962

Bernard Barber, 'Resistance by scientists to scientific discovery', *Science*, vol.134, 1961

Margaret C. Barnet, 'The 1832 cholera epidemic in York', *Medical History*, vol.16, 1972

B.J. Blench, 'The Jersey cholera epidemic of 1832', *Société Jersiaise Annual Bulletin*, vol.19

Asa Briggs, 'Cholera and Society', *Past and Present*, 1961

C. Fraser Brockington, 'The cholera 1831', *The Medical Officer*, vol.96, 1956

———, 'Public health at the Privy Council, 1831-34', *Journal of the History of Medicine*, vol.16, 1961

P.E. Brown, 'John Snow, the autumn loiterer', *Bulletin of the History of Medicine*, vol.35, 1961

S.P.W. Chave, 'Henry Whitehead and the cholera in Broad Street', *Medical History*, vol.11, 1958

———, 'The Broad Street pump and after', *Medical Officer*, vol.99, 1958

Louis Chevalier, *Le Choléra*, Paris, 1958

Charles Creighton, *A History of epidemics*, 2 vols., 2nd edition, London, 1965

Michael Durey, *The first spasmodic cholera epidemic in York*, Borthwick Papers, no.48, York, 1974

Clifford Geertz, 'Religion as a cultural system', in M. Banton (ed.), *Anthropological approaches to religion*, London, 1966

E.D.W. Greig, 'The treatment of cholera by intravenous saline injections; with particular reference to the contributions of Dr Thomas Latta of Leith', *Edinburgh Medical and Surgical Journal*, vol.53, 1946

B. Hamilton, 'The Medical Profession in the 18th century', *Economic History Review*, 2nd series, vol.4 1951

S.W.F. Holloway, 'Medical Education in England, 1830-1858', *History*, vol.49 1964

Thomas S. Kuhn, *The structure of scientific revolutions*, Chicago, 1970

Roderick E. McGrew, *Russia and the cholera, 1823-1832*, Madison, 1965

Alan MacLaren, 'Bourgeois ideology and Victorian philanthropy: the contradictions of cholera', in A.A. MacLaren (ed.), *Social class in Scotland: past and present*, Edinburgh, 1976

N.C. MacNamara, *Asiatic Cholera*, London, 1892

J. MacPherson, *Annals of cholera from the earliest periods to the year 1872*, London, 1872

R.J. Morris, 'Religion and medicine; the cholera pamphlets of Oxford,' *Medical History*, vol.19, 1975

Charles F. Mullett, 'A century of English Quarantine', *Bulletin of the History of Medicine*, vol.23, 1949

R. Pollitzer, *Cholera*, Geneva, 1959

Charles E. Rosenberg, *The cholera years, United States, 1832, 1849 and 1866*, Chicago, 1962

———, 'Cholera in 19th century Europe', *Comparative Studies in Society and History*, vol.8, 1965-66

R.H. Shryock, 'Nineteenth century medicine: scientific aspects,' *Cahier d'histoire Mondiale*, vol.3, 1957

John Stokes, *The history of the cholera epidemic of 1832 in Sheffield*, Sheffield, 1921

S. Swaroop and M.V. Raman, 'The endemicity of cholera in relation to fairs and festivals in India', *Indian Journal of Medical Research*, vol.39, 1941

H.P. Tait, 'The cholera board of health Edinburgh, 1831-34', *Medical Officer*, vol.97, 1957

INDEX

Aberdeen 101
Acland, Dr Thomas 210
Administration 33-5, 50, 51;
  plans 70, 71; structures 71, 73-4,
  205-6; weakness 112
Alarm 17, 43, 55, 64, 67, 98, 116,
  117, 121, 200
Alison, Edward 123, 162, 167, 168
Althorpe, Lord 151
Anatomy 99, 101, 103, 113, 160
  and class 102; fears of in
  Manchester 111
Anglican Church 132, 134, 140,
  145-6, 147, 148
Anti-popery 131, 134, 141, 155
Apathy 27, 55, 85, 93, 117
Apothecary 51, 63
Arthur, James, Deputy Inspector
  General of Hospitals 59, 63, 66,
  67, 68, 69, 96
Artillery against cholera 173
Ashley, Lord 205
Astrakhan 21, 22, 27, 171
Authority 40, 67, 86-7, 154;
  and class 95; and medical skill 26;
  and social prestige 25-6; lack of
  legal by administration 59-60;
  social 33

Backworth 61
Baker, Robert 163, 176, 180, 181,
  186, 189, 191, 197, 199
Baku 22
Baltic 23-4
Baptists 132
Barry, Dr David 25, 32, 33, 34, 50
Beith, Ayrshire 74
Belfast 141
Bell, George Hamilton 15, 64, 115,
  163, 164, 165, 167, 181
Bell ringing 173
Bengal 21, 22
Berlin 84
Bible 131, 140, 141, 152-3
Bilston 16, 106, 119, 122, 123,
  145, 197; and drink 137
Bleeding 163

Blomfield, Bishop of London 148,
  150, 203, 205
Body snatching 101-2, 109-11, 160
Brandy 11
Bread Riots 113
Brewery Workers 138
Bristol 74
British and Foreign Bible Society 141
British Critic 155
Broad Street Pump 208
Broussian School 165, 185
Budd, Dr William 206-7
Bullen, Simeon 59, 62, 67-8
Burial customs of the working
  classes 105-6
Burial Regulations 104-5, 112
Burials 35, 73, 106
Burnett, Sir William, victualling
  office 26
Byam, Sir I., comptroller of the
  navy 26

Calcutta 21
Campsie 67
Canals 66
Carpenter's Political Magazine 27, 34
Castor oil 163
Catholics 145, 147, 154
Central Board of Health 25, 40, 43,
  54, 59, 63, 72-3, 74, 80, 112,
  183, 197-8
Central government weakness 54
Central-local government
  relationships 40, 41, 43, 44, 47-54,
  68-9, 73
Chadwick, Edwin 34, 200, 202
Chalmers, Thomas 131
Cheltenham 118
Chemistry 165, 166, 190
Chester 74
Chetney Hill 24
China 21
Cholera Act 72, 150, 203
Christian Observer 132, 133, 153
Church and King 98, 145
Circulars 67, 71
Circulars from Board of Health 33

222

Index

Clanny, Dr Reid 11, 39, 41, 44, 45, 49, 171-2, 176
Class and drink 136
Class relationships 17, 189-90
Cleansing 35, 60, 73, 107, 141, 174-5, 206
Cleland, James 81
Clergy 33, 51, 62, 68, 89, 146, 154, 186, 187, 197, 209
Clerkenwell ballad 96
Clinical history 14, 15
Coal interests 46, 47, 51, 53, 60
Cobbett, William 96, 107, 120, 149
Coercion 31-2, 33, 35, 112, 113
Colliers 61, 89
Commercial interests 32, 51; and quarantine 24
Community studies 186-90
Congregationalists 132, 134, 139, 140, 141, 154
Contact, means of 65
Contagion, see miasma-contagion debate
Covenanter 134
Cowan, Dr Robert 81
Creagh, Lt. Col. 44
Creighton, Charles 197
Crisis reaction 14
Cromarty Bay 24
Cromarty Reform Bill meeting 125
Customs 24, 41

Darwin 130
Daun, Dr 43, 44, 50, 51, 55, 59, 61, 113
De Jonnes, M Moreau 22
Death rates 12, 75, 81, 82, 160; age specific 81, 82, 83; cholera 13, 27; class differentials 87-92; Edinburgh 81-3; European 84; Gateshead 62; Glasgow 67, 81-3; India 22; Newburn 62; Sunderland 55
Dehydration effects 15, 165
Denial of cholera 45, 48, 49-50, 60, 61, 70
Descartes 130, 147
Destruction of clothes of the poor 107
Diarrhoea 11, 12
Diet 35, 174
Dirt and disease 34
Disaster studies 18
Dissections 44

Dodd, Henry 161, 163-4, 174-5, 181
Doherty, John 96, 160; and anatomists 111
Drainage and cholera 60, 61, 119
Drink 15, 34, 64, 65, 66, 80, 85, 86, 100, 110, 115, 116, 118-9, 133, 134-7, 155, 174-5, 182, 186, 187, 198; the clinical link with cholera 138
Dumfries 123, 162, 179, 206
Duncan, Dr 200

East Lothian villages 65
Edinburgh 64, 65-6, 81, 115, 117, 118, 138, 141, 159, 167-70, 175-6; riots 108-9
Edinburgh Medical and Surgical Journal 34, 46, 165-8, 182
Electricity 171, 190-1
Embleton parish surgeon 40, 51
Evangelicals 131-4, 139-42, 143, 150, 153-4; and death 140; and miasma 182-3
Exeter 74, 106, 146, 173, 175
Expectations 18, 19, 48, 93, 97, 103, 114, 160, 198, 200, 201
Expenses 69
Explanations 177-8
Eyam plague deaths 14

Fairs 65, 74, 115, 116, 118-9; Bilston wakes week 119; St Giles Fair Oxford 119
Family and cholera 32, 82, 104
Farr, William 215
Fast day 147-51, 202
Fear and help for the poor 120-21
Fee paying and medical men 39, 45, 54, 63, 160, 161-2
Filth and cholera 60, 62, 64, 67, 85, 111, 171, 175, 180, 187, 197, 199
Finance 72, 73, 74
First cases 42, 43, 48, 54, 55, 64, 65, 67
Flax and the flax trade 23, 24, 29, 54
Flitting day, Glasgow 118-19
Friendly societies 106, 160
Fumigation 173, 174
Fungus theory 207-8

Galvanism 165, 190
Ganges 22

Gateshead 16, 62; Bottle Bank 134, 137; revival 145
Gaulter, Henry 111, 171, 178, 180, 181, 186, 189-90, 191, 197
General Board of Health 201, 202, 205-6, 209
Geographical segregation of social classes 52, 84, 124
Geology and religion 130-1
Gibralter Yellow Fever 25
Gibson, Dr of Edinburgh 50, 51, 62, 63
Girdlestone, Rev. Charles 186, 199; and drink 137
Glasgow 55, 56, 67, 81, 83, 100, 138, 159, 161, 178, 179, 200; flitting day 118-19; riots 109
God of battles 202
God of the gaps 161, 204
God the avenger 151-2, 154, 204
God the reformer 204
God the scientist 131
Goosedubbs, Glasgow 67
Green vegetables and infection 15
Greville, Charles 23, 24, 25, 32, 86

Haddington 64, 66, 71, 80, 179
Half pay military men 59, 64
Halford, Sir Henry 25, 33, 34
Hamburg 23, 27
Hamilton, Duke of 67
Handbills 64, 96, 115-6
Hastings, Army of the Marquis of 21
Hastings, Charles 161
Hawick 65
Hawkers 66
Helplessness of medical men 22
Hetton 61
Hindu Kush 23
Holland, Henry 26
Holland, John, poet and journalist 144
Hood, Thomas 99
Hospitals 39, 33-4, 42, 49, 51, 62, 63, 64, 67, 69, 73, 80, 103, 104, 112, 115, 116, 125, 141, 161, 172, 173, 183, 189; and rioting 108-17; fear of 103
Hot air bath 164
Houghton-le-Spring 61, 62, 161, 163, 171, 181
House-to-house visitations 107
Hull 55
Humbug 96, 97-8, 109
Hume, David 178

Hume, Joseph 27, 30, 33, 70, 97
Humoral pathology 163
Hunt, Henry 70
Hurdwar 21, 22
Huxley 130

Ideologues 165, 185
Idolatry 134, 139
Incomes 87
India 21, 22
Indian Medical men 15, 163, 171, 181
Infection and burials 106
Information 201
Information,search for 24, 39, 51, 59, 68-9, 71, 72
Internal quarantine 53, 118
Internal trade, India 21
Irish 131, 176; and burials 105 and riots 111-2
Irish famine 12, 200
Irvine 68
Irvingites 150

Jedburgh 14
Jessore 21
Jobbery 97

Kay, Dr James 85, 186, 197, 200
Keelmen 11, 42, 46, 60
Kell, James Butler 11, 39, 41, 42, 43, 44
Kendal 187
Keswick 27, 119, 148
Kilwinning 68
Kirghiz Steppe 23
Kirk 132
Kirkintilloch 66, 67, 179
Kock, Robert 15, 209
Kuhn, Thomas 176

Lancet 25, 26, 34, 46, 161, 182
Latta, Dr Thomas 165, 166-70, 185, 189, 190, 214
Law-giving mob 111-13
Leeds 117, 119-20, 163, 175, 176, 180, 181, 186, 189, 199, 200
Legal authority 71, 73
Legitimate rights 93
Leigh, Rev. William of Bilston 106, 147, 186; and drink 137
Leith 79

Index

Lemington 61
Levant Company 24
Lightning 172, 176, 190
Lincoln 74
Literacy 116
Liverpool 72, 200; merchants 24; Methodist conference 143; Reform Bill meeting 124-5
Local Boards of Health 31, 33-5, 53, 71, 73, 74, 173; Edinburgh 64; Edinburgh handbills 115; Glasgow 66; Irvine 69; Leeds 119; Newcastle 60; Oxford handbills 115-16; Rotherhithe 70; Sheffield 119; Sunderland 39, 43, 50, 51; and medical men 117
Lodging-houses 65, 73
London 30, 70, 206; death rates 12
London Gazette 25
Londonderry, Lord 47, 53, 86
Lovett 100

MacCann, Francis 62
MacDonald, Major R. 32, 64
MacLean, London physician 24
MacLean, William 32
MacMichael, William 26
MacNamara 15
Magistrates 33, 39, 42, 130
Malthus 99
Manchester 30, 85-6, 99, 103, 131, 33-5, 53, 71, 179, 180, 181, 186, 189, 197, 200, 201; Board of Health 1790, 31; riots, Swan Street Hospital 110-11
Markets 65, 74, 116, 118-19
Marriage and cholera 144
Marshall, John, Leeds flax manufacturer 29, 87
Marshall, Lt. Colonel John 32
Maton, Dr William George 26
Mauritius 11, 39, 179
McGrigor, Sir James, Army hospitals 26, 40, 43
Mead, Dr Richard 23, 172, 183
Medical profession 33, 34, 39, 40, 42, 45, 48, 51, 54, 67-9, 80, 98, 101-3, 123, 159-92, 201; and social pressures 24; distrust and hostility 160-2; distrust of hampers research 190; popular resistance to 99, 108-17; social structure 159-60
Medical research 161, 166-70
Medical topography 186-91
Medway 24
Melbourne, Lord 47, 86
Miasma-contagion 25, 28, 31, 35, 40, 44, 49-50, 66, 121, 129, 170-84, 206-9
Miasma-contagion debate 1848 202
Microscope 160, 192, 206-7
Middle classes 80, 86, 87, 91-3, 95, 117-25, 131, 136, 150, 160, 162, 179, 197, 202, 208; and religion 144; fear of cholera 95; fear of disease 86; fear of working class as disease source 117-18; flight 122-4; perception of the working class 93, 95, 100; and the miasma-contagion debate 182-4
Military cordons, Prussia and Russia, 23
Miller, Hugh 202
Mining 65, 145, 171
Mining villages 68
Miracles 130, 142
Monistic pathologies 164, 166, 177
Montgomery, James, poet and journalist 119, 124, 144, 213
Moral assumptions 93
Moral influence on science 182
Moral response to disease 129-55, 213-14
Morals and cholera 17, 186, 198, 199
Moscow 23, 24, 84, 112
Musselburgh 65, 66, 174, 179

Naval blockade of Sunderland 45
Neale, Dr Adam 170, 171-2, 185, 191
Newburn 16, 62, 145, 189; victims' occupations 89; death rate 12
Newcastle 44, 59-62, 65, 70, 80, 116, 132, 135, 144, 179, 181; drink to keep cholera away 100; shipping interests 30
Newspaper stamp duties 96
Nijni Novgorod 23
Nineveh 153, 204
North Shields 61, 179
Nurses 42, 89, 90, 179

O'Shaughnessy 165, 166-70, 190
Occupational classification 87-8

226 Index

Occupations of victims 40, 42, 79-92, 188, 189
Old Handsel Monday 65, 118
Opium 11, 80, 162, 164, 165
Opposition to medical profession 67-9
Order in Council 73
Orenburg 23
Oxford 79, 104, 113, 117, 118, 119, 173, 186, 199, 200; occupations of victims 90, 91

Paisley 109-10
Paley 130
Palmerston 214
Panic 18, 122
Paradigms and cholera 176-7, 215
Parliamentary debates 27, 70, 150-1, 204-5
Parliamentary reform as diversion from cholera 96, 98
Paternalism 52, 53, 86, 112-13, 146; and middle class 119
Pentecostalism 150
Perceval, Spencer 149, 150-1
Persia 21
Phillpotts, Bishop of Exeter 146
Physicians, Royal College of 24, 25, 26, 28, 29, 32
Pickwick Papers 136
Pig Sties 61, 73, 176
Pilgrims 22
Pilots 40, 41
Plague 12, 13, 23, 27, 29, 172
Plague 1720 24
Poland 23
Poor Law 71-3, 74, 83, 99, 118, 162, 198, 206
Ports and cholera 119
Post-mortems 80, 113, 185
Poulett-Thompson 30, 53, 70, 148
Poverty 51, 63, 80, 98, 148, 186, 197, 198, 204; and cholera 133, and morality 65
Poverty theory of cholera 35, 49, 65, 84-6, 120
Poverty theory of cholera from working-class radicals 100
Prayer 140-3, 145, 146-7, 202-3
Pre-disposing causes 174-5
Preparations, Sunderland 41
Presbyterians 134, 140, 153, 155, 203
Presidency reports 22

Press reaction 14, 21, 27, 34, 43, 44, 48, 85, 137
Prestonpans 65
Privy Council 23, 24, 29, 32
Prostitutes 80, 111, 199
Proudfoot, Thomas 187
Public Health Acts 1848 204-6
Public health reform 17
Purgatives 163, 202
Pyn, Sir William 23, 24, 32, 47, 81

Quarantine 17, 23, 24, 25, 28, 29, 33, 35, 53, 54, 55, 59, 61, 71, 172, 179, 183, 214-5; blamed for famine and unemployment 30; opposition to 30, 50, 53; opposition to by Sunderland commercial interests 45; regulations 41, 44; opposition to regulations 47; reaction to regulations and their influence on the flax trade 29
Quarterly Review 14
Quekett 185, 207

Radicals 95, 97, 98, 99, 133; and drink 138; and God 150; and medical men 160; and miasma-contagion debate 183, and religion 130; and the fast day 148-9
Reform agitation 124
Reform Bill crisis 47, 133
Registrar-General 12, 201, 209-10
Regulations 103, 147
Relative visiting 66
Religion and cholera 198, 202-4
Religion and disease 213-4
Religion and medicine 191
Religion and science 129-31, 139-40, 142-3, 170, 172, 182-3
Religious symbolism 151-3
Research 69, 178, 189-90, 191 206-7
Resistance to new ideas 167-70
Resources and action 18
Revivals, religious 144-5, 203
Rice water evacuations 15
Riga 23
Riots 27, 46, 47, 86, 98, 101, 106, 108-17, 160
Riots in Europe 112
Royal College of Physicians 182, 183, 202
Ruling class 27, 47, 52, 53, 86,

Index

87, 147, 153-4, 197; and contagion n 183; response to the mob 112-3
Russell 34

Saline infusion 165, 166-70, 189
Salisbury 12
Sandgate 62
Science and social pressure 17, 180-1 183-4, 202, 209, 214-5
Scientific community 177-8, 191-2
Scientific understanding 129
Scotland 59, 73, 74; finance difficulties 72, riots 108-10
Seaham Harbour 47
Secession churches, Scotland 132
Secondary causes 146
Seghill 61
Seymour, Edward 26
Sharp, Sir Cuthbert, Collector of Customs at Sunderland 41
Sheffield 119, 144, 206, 213
Shipping interests 51; in Sunderland 45
Shock disease 14
Simon, Sir John 197, 209
Sin and disease 132-5, 140-2, 147, 153-4, 155, 203
Smallpox 14, 172, 198
Snow, Dr John 207-10, 214
Social class 52, 53, 65, 80, 83-93, 95-126
Social policy and cholera 198
Social pressure and science 50, 172-3
Social pressure on the medical profession 46, 48, 51
Social status 40
Social status and belief 153-4
Social structure of Sunderland 52
Solly, Henry 121, 124
Southey, Robert 27, 98, 119, 148
Spasms after death 106-7
Sproat, William 11, 42
St Petersburg 25
Stability, social 17, 114, 125-6, 145, 147
Standgate Creek 24
Stark, James 81
Statistics 17, 22, 75, 81, 185-6, 187-90, 191, 202, 207-10
Status and the medical profession 192, 207-8
Status, social 26, 167-70, 182
Stereotypes of victims 85-6

Stewart, Edward, Deputy Chairman of the Navy Board 26, 32
Stockton 53
Sunderland 11, 39-56, 59, 60, 104, 115, 134, 139, 171, 176, 179, 181, 186, 187-8, 197; victims' occupations 88
Surgeons 11, 39, 40, 88, 89, 90, 159
Surgeons, India, contagion beliefs 28
Swalwell 61
Sydenham 164, 186
Symptoms 11, 15, 16, 34, 40, 49-50, 60, 164, 207

Tar barrels 173
Tehran 22
Test of society 17, 74, 213
Textile manufacturers 46
The moral and physical condition of the working classes 85
Theology 17
Tipton 119, 145
Topaz 179
Trade routes and cholera 23, 25
Trades unions 96
Tranent 65, 66
Treasury 69
Treatments 11, 34, 35, 80, 162-6, 185-6, 187-90, 201
Troop cordons in Britain 33; in Russia 28
Troop movements, India 21
Troops and riots 109-12, 114
Turner, Dr Thomas 26
Typhus 12, 100, 205

Unitarians 142-3, 148, 153

Vagrants 61-2, 65, 66, 71, 89, 117-8
Values and action 17, 18, 95
Vaughan connection 25
Vaughan, Thomas 186
Vegetables 175
Volga River 22
Voluntary subscriptions 39, 44, 53, 119, 121

Wages 87
Wakeley, Thomas 161
Walker, British physician in Moscow 24
Wallposters 115-16
Warburton 27
Warner, Peleham 26

Warsaw 84
Water supply 16, 61, 62, 71, 138, 187, 197, 206, 207-9, 215
Weavers book of weft 149
Wednesbury 74
Wesleyan Methodists 15, 132, 133, 134-5, 140, 143, 144, 153, 154, 155, 186, 203
Westminster Medical Society 70, 180, 181

Whitewash 107, 173, 174
Wide Open 61
Williamson, Sir Hedworth 46
Woollen Trade 29
Working-class distrust of Boards of Health 117
Working-class reaction 100

Yarmouth 12
Yellow fever 23, 25, 50

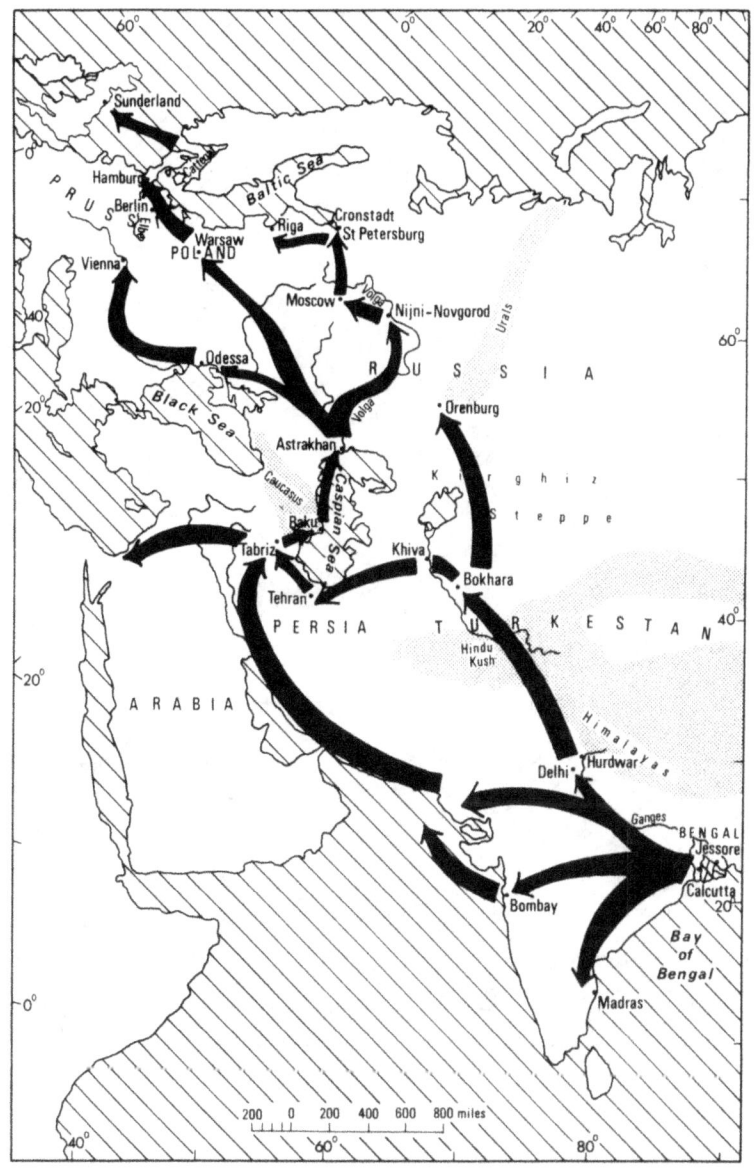

Map one: Bengal to Sunderland, 1826-1831

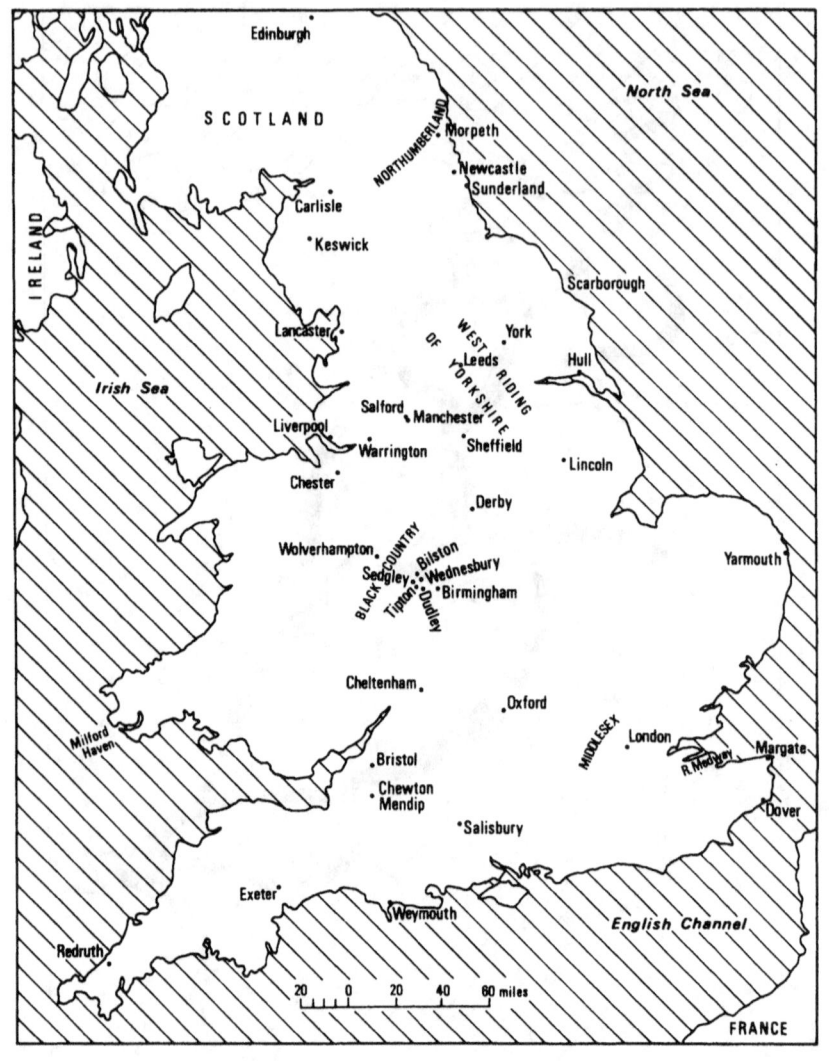

Map two: England and Wales, 1831-1832

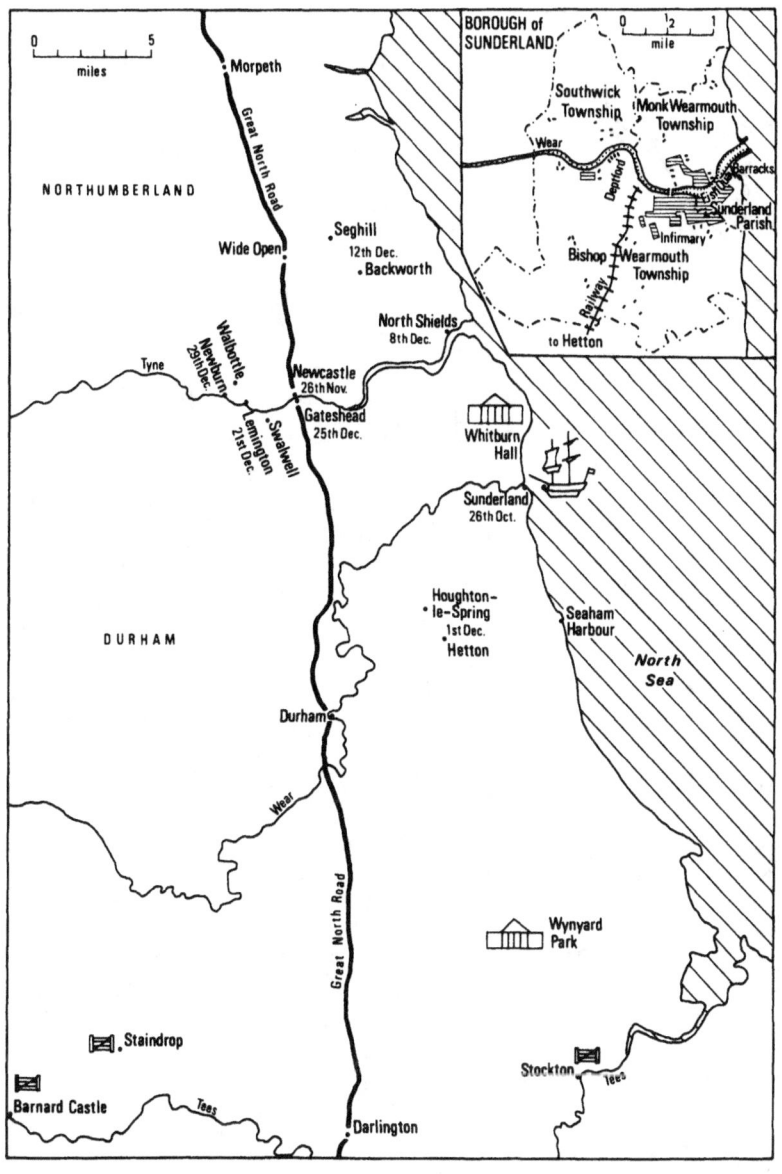

Map three: North-East England, winter 1831-1832. The gates show those places which attempted to blockade the Sunderland road. Dates are given for the first case of cholera.

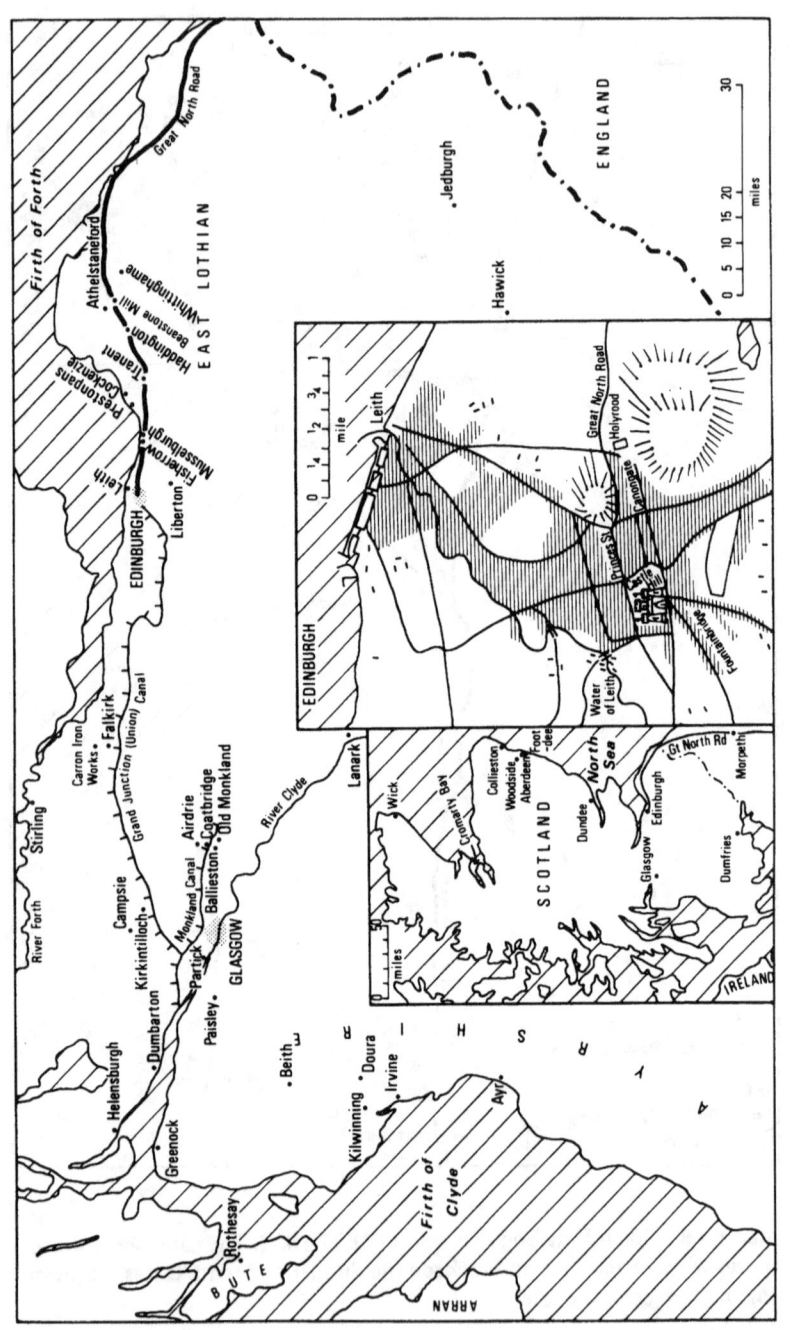

Map four: Scotland, 1831-32

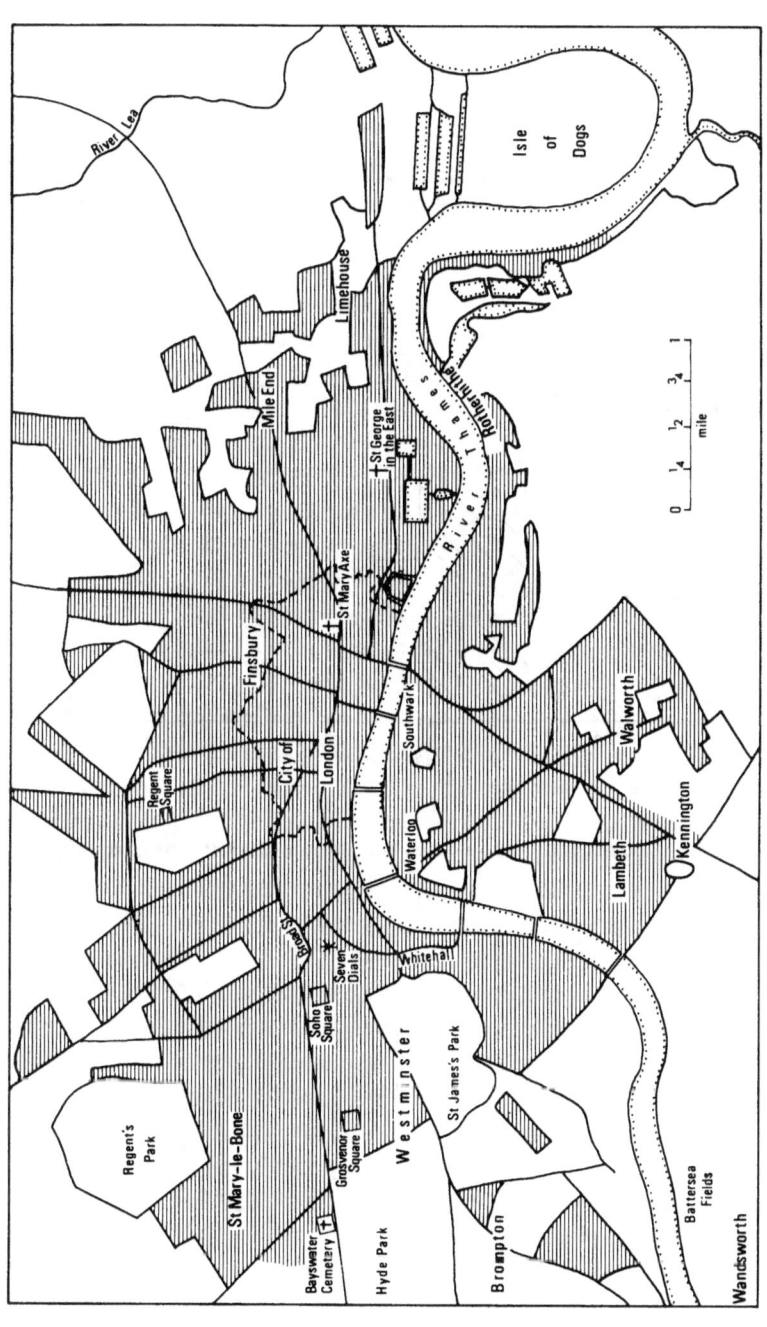

Map five: London 1832-1866. Although the built up area indicated applies to 1832, several names relevant to the later epidemics have been added.

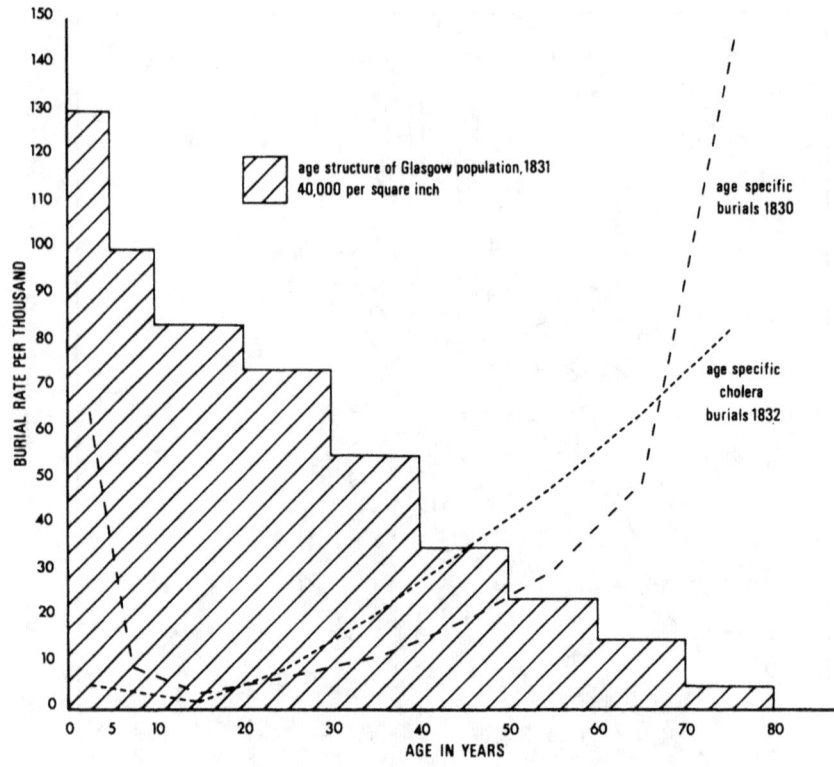

Figure one: Age-specific burial rates and the age structure of Glasgow, 1830-1831

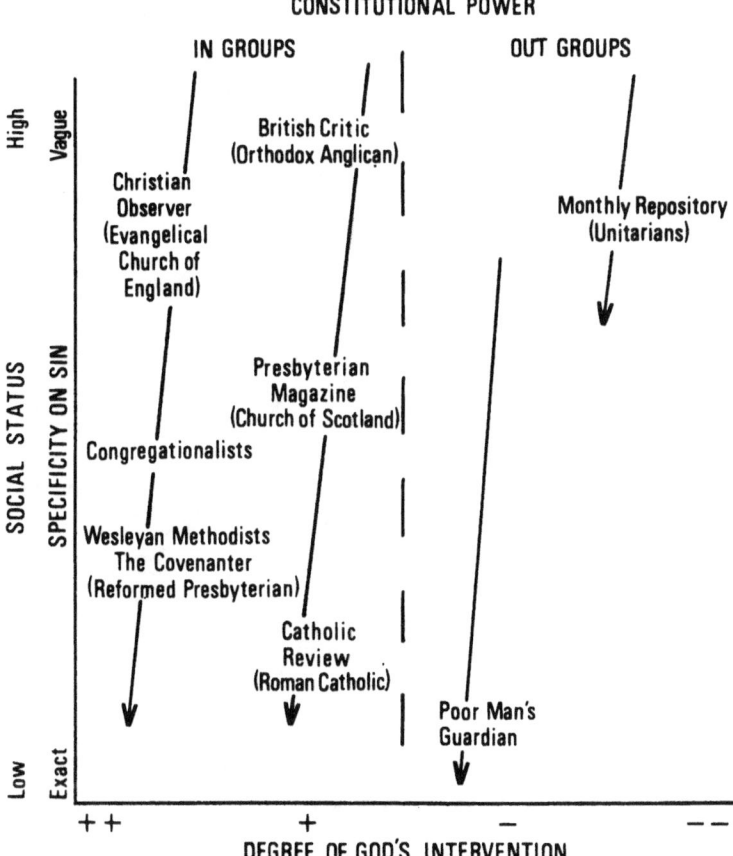

Figure two: Religion, cholera and social status, 1832

For Product Safety Concerns and Information please contact our EU representative GPSR@taylorandfrancis.com
Taylor & Francis Verlag GmbH, Kaufingerstraße 24, 80331 München, Germany

www.ingramcontent.com/pod-product-compliance
Lightning Source LLC
Chambersburg PA
CBHW062216300426
44115CB00012BA/2090